I0425032

The
Top 25 Things
You Can Do To Change
Your Life
For the Better...Forever

by

GSIMMS

--Forward--

When answering the question of why I wrote this book, the answer was easy, immediate and two-fold.

> · *Knowing what I learned from personal experience, I can help you if you are having health challenges, and*
> · *If you want to avoid health problems, I can help you by making accurate information available to you so that you can make better choices.*

For the past 20-plus months, "Health and Wellness" has been more than a passion or pre-occupation for me. Health and Wellness has been a way of life because this has been the core of my recovery from a heart related health crisis that totally blind sided me. In fact, while laying in the hospital (some 24 days), I had much to consider. I decided that if I were allowed to walk out of there, I'd use my divinely given talent as a writer/communicator to create a work that might benefit those who desperately need it.

As a result, this book, "Volume I—The Top 25 Things You Can Do to Change Your Life For the Better...Forever" was born along with , GSimms-HealthandWellness.com, and FYI-HealthandWellness.blogspot.com.

The mission is simple–publish good information that will help you make better choices.

I know that there are a host of other sites and books written about Health and Wellness.

But considering that, this book is different because it represents what I've discovered to work as a result of personal experience. I walk this walk daily as my personal prescription to living in a wholesome manner. I stand behind every word written and every suggestion made. In other words, this book, in many ways, is a copy of my diary for healthy living.

So, thank you for allowing me to share.

I would be remiss in not saying also that there are many people in my life who have and continue to touch and inspire me in ways that I could never repay. For this work, however, I'll just name two—my mom, Rose, and my daughter, Portia. And to the many others, but especially to "my girl"–*The Inimitable Dove*, I say thank you.

For my younger audience, pay attention. Learn from what you are seeing and reading. Digest the information. As you learn something of value, make modifications to your path in support of a journey that will assuredly point you in the direction of "conscious choices' about something that we all have paid too little attention to—our health.

Do enjoy and let me know how you're feeling.

G Simms

Table of Contents

About the Author

It pays to understand a bit about Gary Simms' background and life experience to truly appreciate his quick direct wit, and oft times profoundly introspective reflections.

He was born into a middle-class family in New Orleans, Louisiana during the mid-1950's. GSimms (his pen name) draws from the focus and discipline of a star youth athlete, the intelligence of a summa cum laude graduate of his college class, the sophistication of an Environmental Communications Executive for a Fortune 100 company, and the savvy of a shrewd businessman/entrepreneur to render unexpected essence and flavor with a unique filter for life and quality living.

Passionate and driven to succeed, Simms has taken what he describes as "one of my very dark personal moments," to fashion a work that he hopes will contribute significantly to the lives of those wanting to be better and do better.

"When most people discuss achievement and improvement, the goal is oft times for external manifestation," says Simms, while gazing off and collecting his thoughts. "I am fervent about this and say that the focus should always be internal. You have to improve inside to truly reflect improvement outwardly. You have to be better and when you are, the world will see it."

His passion has become the enthusiastic pursuit of life, health and wellness. "Far too many people suffer through less than a great quality of life due to relinquishing their life responsibility to everyone else--the so-called authorities, media news bites, so-called experts, doctors, etc.," he says. "I believe the pathway to restoration begins with owning information that is accurate, understandable, and readily accessible."

GSimms' valued quips, thoughts, humor and advice is peppered throughout his blogs, articles, podcasts, speeches, presentations, and conversations.

Look for more from GSimms. He plans to continue his work as a health and wellness writer and currently publishes GSimms-HealthandWellness.com, GSimms-TheTop25.com, and http://FYI-HealthandWellness.blogspot.com.

Additionally, he's working on two books that tell of his Hurricane Katrina experiences.

About the Author

When recently asked to consider developing a site for his unique brand of funny, serious and always insightful social commentary, he responded, "Oh...I will probably have to because we've chosen a collective position of numbness about lots of things that somebody should say something about."

We can't wait.

And finally, stay tuned for his first novel--a love story that twists and turns in a way that could only be fictional...but perhaps not.

Known for being a "real character" to his close friends, GSimms relishes entertainment yet appreciates his reading and listening audience and respects his platform to inform.

GSimms' Tribe

As Presented...

The text of this book is organized specifically to address matters that impact the mind, body, and soul.

Without delivering an esoteric speech here, these three entities represent the essence of every man...as we see him moving about us in one embodiment.

With that in mind, I've organized the chapters under those flags...Mind, Body and Soul.

As you will note in reading this book, the tips or chapters under Soul could easily go under the Mind flag; however, for me those chapters represent a deeper core and therefore are best represented under Soul.

It is my intent that you might find jewels that you can apply to your life.

I would recommend that you make an attempt to apply the strategies of this book in stages. I can't imagine overwhelming yourself with all 25 tips at once. Keep your copy handy and use it as a reference.

Thank you so much for allowing me to share this opportunity and information.

GSimms
GSimms.com

MIND

TIP No. 1

Focus

Focus is a challenge for most people and represents one of the major reasons why most people feel unfulfilled and are ultimately unsuccessful.

What I mean by this is really simple. Most people have a problem keeping their eye on the prize (whatever represents the prize for them). In fact, many can't answer a direct question about their goals. When faced with that question, you're likely to get showered with a speech about everything other than what you asked. For instance, you're likely to find out, with emotional specifics, the laundry list of those things that they don't want.

Here's a tip—focus on what you want…not what you don't want.

Okay, you say that you're not getting it. So the deal here is that you don't know how to focus. Maybe you're accustomed to just winging it or doing what you do as it comes. If your way is one of random acts of whatever, let me take a minute to help you out.

First and foremost focus has to do with concentration, operating a clear and distinct plan to fruition, and moving forward on your plan with laser sharp and unwavering commitment.

Now, having said that, you must understand that everybody and everything will surface as a distraction to your goal; however, those distractions or obstacles are the reason you need to learn the skill of focusing.

Still need help? Try the following tips on for size.

- **Keep going past your frustration, tiredness or willingness to give up**
  I've often heard coaches and mentors say to their students that "success is right there for you to have if you just hang in there." Over the years as both an athlete and businessman I agree. Many times the difference in a win or loss is your willingness to do just 'one more'.

- **Multi-Tasking is your enemy**
  If you are going to really get stuff done, you should think seriously about learning how to direct your energies and thoughts so that you can handle the job at hand—one task/thought at a time. If you have several things to do, prioritize them and commit dedicated energy to each until you have done as much as you can with that task. By listing your items, you don't have to commit any brain cells or energy to them until you've gotten to that task on your list.

Focus

- **Overcome putting off the inevitable (yep, overcome procrastination)**
  Let's be real here. It's probably easier to do it now than to suffer through not doing whatever it is that you're running away from. Can't you hear your mother (or worse, a nagging spouse) grilling you about not having done this, that, or the other. If the task is something that needs doing, do it. Ask yourself if it would be better to do it than to worry about not doing it. Finally, understand that the task won't be easier to do later. As the NIKE commercial says, 'Just Do It'!

- **Ever heard of walking with blinders on?**
  You can play a trick on your brain to force yourself to concentrate. When working on a task, use your hands as blinders or blinkers by cupping them to the sides of your eyes and making a tunnel—hence tunnel vision. This physical ritual will remove other visual stimulation from your eyesight and force you to deal with the information that's before you. In other words, you narrow your vision and focus or concentrate on limited information.

- **Acknowledge what's really important**
  Many times, we spend lots of time drowning ourselves in the stuff that we are expected to see as important (like all of the job related stuff, meetings for organizations that you belong to and the various external opinions that we work so hard to support and validated). By remembering that most of what we value is only important in accordance with perspective, we might take a little more time to rearrange our priorities and view things for what their truly worth. Done with care, you might find the treasured value of your family and personal relationships take on new meaning.

In summary, it's good to understand that focus will enable your ability to achieve at a more fulfilling level. If you are not accustomed to planning and thinking this way, just know that it's never too late to start.

Adopt the practice of focus in every aspect of your life. Concentrate on what you want as it relates to your health, your diet, your emotional well being, your wealth or wealth accumulation, your relationships, your wellness, your fitness, etc. It pays to be specific and remember that focus is not a sprint. You must endorse it as a part of your lifestyle.

RESOURCES/TOOLS FOR YOU TO USE

I fully understand this problem. In fact, I have not always had the focus that I have now. In talking with many people, I also understand that part of the problem might be that you aren't organized as well. So, please accept this gift that I have for you. Log in to this site (www.simpleology.com). It's free. You will start your transformation and become organized while getting laser sharp focus.

TIP No. 2

If What You Do For Work Is Not Your Passion, Find Your Passion and Do That!!!

It's said that water seeks its own level and electricity seeks to complete a circuit. I say that those statements are akin to having the innate desire to be the authentic person that you are.

Very few of us come into the world so abundantly blessed with assets that we never have to work. Most of our existence on this planet will be tied to earning money to sustain ourselves. And since that is the case, you should do everything possible to engage in the kind of work that agrees with your spirit and soul.

A very special woman in my life recently shared something with me that represents the best way I know to articulate this. We were talking about our fathers (both of whom have passed on) and she said that her father told her (in his wisdom) that, at the end of the day, everyone should have had at least three things in their lives:

    A. Meaningful work;
    B. Something to look forward to; and
    C. Someone to love and be loved by

For the purpose of this segment, I'll just deal with the first item—meaningful work.

We have all been blessed with talents—those natural gifts that were planted in us through divine providence. Allow yourself to find your joy, work your joy and subsequently remove the title job from your work.

Studies indicate that more than 65% of the stress that we live with comes from what we do everyday from 9 to 5 (the job).

If you know what your passion is but don't see the opportunity to earn a living from it, your mission (if you choose to accept it) is to create a way to earn a living from your passion.

If you do, your life stresses can be reduced and your life's quality can increase.

As Work: Do What You're Passionate About

RESOURCES/TOOLS FOR YOU TO USE

Understanding what you're truly good at is more difficult than most would imagine. The reason is simple. Each of us has the tendency to either over compensate or under compensate for our personal traits and talents. We will often disregard important tidbits of information when making self evaluations and more often than not ultimately rely on someone else to tell us what they think we're good at. We normally adopt that notion as authentic whether or not it's an accurate assessment.

Rather than do that, I strongly recommend that you purchase the book "Strength Finder 2.0" by Tom Rath.

You can use the link below to do that. I strongly recommend this for a very simple reason. If you learn enough from this exercise to ultimately do what you're good at, your life will become easier and less stressful. I remember my early life as an athlete. People would often tell me that I made playing the game of baseball look easy and fun. Duh...it was for me. My point is, if you're doing what you're good at, it is as easy for you as it looks to others. To that, I say, don't take your skills for granted...don't live another day without doing an objective exercise that will answer the questions without any doubt. The link is here: http://astore.amazon.com/gsimmshealth-20

TIP No. 3

Learn How To Manage or Eliminate Stress From Your Life

As a writer, I read volumes of information—especially information that pertains to my area of interest and specialization—Health and Wellness.

As a result, I had the good fortune of reading a good article written by Lucy Danzinger of Self.com. It was entitled, "Stress is Sabotaging your Diet Success."

Well, that is a true statement, but I'm going to take this just a little further. Stress is Sabotaging your health and wellness. In fact, stress proliferates our lives like an epidemic germ that spreads to every cell of our bodies. If left unchecked or uncontrolled, the ravages deplete us of our life source. If you never find a way to manage it correctly, it will suck all appearances of "quality of life" from you.

Do I have your attention?

Let's face it. As of this writing, we are living in a very stressful time. The world economy is in the pits. Unemployment figures are at the highest ever recorded in this country. Even if you have a job, you probably wish that you could make it without the one that you have. Parents are worried and wonder about all sorts of things related to their children. Grown sons and daughters of aging parents are worried about them.

Your mounting stresses wreck havoc on all of your body systems and functions. It causes unnecessary spikes to your blood sugar levels, raises blood pressure, causes you to sleep fewer hours, causes you to eat more, causes headaches, stomach aches, back pain, and makes you a candidate for long term disease.

So how do you handle stress?

If your situation doesn't lend itself to your being able to eliminate the source of your stress, you need to take steps to effectively manage it. Here are a few tips that work.

MUSIC. Listen to music that inspires you. Listen to music that you truly enjoy…the music that makes you sing along, tap your feet and makes you want to dance or relax. Here's a stretch. Like to sing. Check out www.singsnap.com. You can sing karaoke online. It's all about having fun and participating in something that you'll enjoy. Check me out on that site at GSimms.

MOVE YOUR BODY. An exercise session is like a magic wand against stress. Just 30 minutes will release a battalion of nature's stress fighting chemicals in your body. It's truly like magic. Choose something that you truly enjoy and let the sweat roll.

Learn How to Manage or Eliminate Stress

HAVE A HEARTY LAUGH. Do you have a friend that makes you laugh? Call him or her. Enjoy the moment. Laughter does your body good. It's like a one-two punch against stress when combined with exercise.

TALK IT OUT. You've got to be careful with this one. Throwing a pity party and inviting others into it IS NOT THE SUGGESTION HERE. Call or visit someone that is level headed and open minded. This person should also be a proactive thinker. Discuss the stressful situation briefly by addressing it and how it makes you feel. After getting those preliminaries out of the way, brainstorm ways that you can resolve or solve the stressful issue and move forward.

TREAT OR PAMPER YOURSELF. You've got to be careful with this one also. Don't use this tip as an excuse for why you spent money that you didn't have. Find an inexpensive indulgence and enjoy the moment. Suggestions include: Take a relaxing bath and engulf your senses with aromatic scented candles or bath salts. Top that off with a deep breathing session for 10 minutes. You will activate neurons and stimulate the release of serotonin—in this case, your secret agents that will help you beat that stress away.

ENJOY A MOMENT AT THE PARK. Weather permitting, go to the park and enjoy the ducks by the pond or spend a few moments walking barefoot on the grass. According to "The Complete Guide to Natural Healing," walking barefoot on grass is a therapeutic form of foot massage (reflexology) that benefits the entire body. According to various studies, walking barefoot on grass is known to support or correct standing posture and has been used to treat insomnia.

REVISIT A FOND OR EXCITING MEMORY. This is like having a moment with yourself that was very special to you. Sounds a little quirky, but never-the-less, this is good medicine. Reflect on that special moment or activity. Recall how you felt, what you saw...the colors...the setting...the temperature...those that you shared the moment with...the excitement or peacefulness of the moment. Close your eyes and hold onto that for as long as it makes sense to. Open your eyes, take a deep breath. The result of this voids tension and stress while lowering blood pressure.

KEEP A JOURNAL. The "Journal of Health Psychology" did a study that revealed that a month of expressive writing can help reduce hypertension. So, write it out. In a way, it allows you to step outside of your direct attachment to the stressor and perform the task of journaling it. In doing so, you can look at the stressor with more logic and find pathways for dealing with the anxiety and the other impacts.

Learn How to Manage or Eliminate Stress

SHARE A LITTLE LOVE. Hopefully your sweetie or significant other is not the source of your stress. That being said, a good full on hug or a passionate kiss can increase endorphin levels while having sex is known to have the greatest effect at de-stressing the body.

LEND A HELPING HAND. Research has proven that scenarios where you are freely giving or teaching can create warm human encounters. Those connections foster an environment that enables your body to function at reduced stress levels.

TIP No. 4

Learn the Skills of Relaxation

Because there are so many people who don't have a lot of experience having felt just how interconnected our minds and bodies are, I decided to expand upon Tip No. 3 Learn How to Manage or Eliminate Stress from your Life.

Without question, relaxation is the result of executing a skill set that pays tremendous benefits to the human spirit and experience.

I've personally witnessed innumerable situations where individuals have placed themselves in personal peril because they simply refuse to relax or don't know how.

One story that comes to mind is that of a man who for the life of himself just does not have the capacity to relax. Considering that this situation is one that I've personally witnessed, I can only convey that I feel sorry for someone who suffers this plight.

This man's behavior is characterized by impatience, being fidgety about almost everything, and always being in a rush (especially when there is no motivation to rush).

If any of that sounds familiar, slow down…take a deep breath…chill out.

Okay, you can say that to some people and they will, but it's obvious that for some, this is easier said than done.

If you'd examine what this kind of existence does to your health, it pays dividends to remove yourself from the tether of that time bomb.

Whether that behavior is the product of a person's inability to handle stress well or whether it is a statement of individual personality, the condition can and should be studied and examined by someone trained in that area. This does not represent a presentation of those findings. The intent here is merely to identify a behavior and address it from a perspective that could help you if you think about this for a minute. Many of us unconsciously create stresses that can be avoided. Additionally, we make matters worse by reacting poorly to our stresses–some to the extent that we eventually desensitize ourselves to natural ways of dealing effectively with them.

There are hundreds of causes of those conditions that produce the kinds of stress that will cause you to desperately need immediate relaxation.

Learn the Skills of Relaxation

If you do not learn to control your stressors, you'll react in a negative manner emotionally and physically. Such maladies as anxiety, being fatigued, being temperamental, finding it hard to breathe, experiencing chest pains, not being to sleep or sleeping excessively can all be signs of needing to simply relax.

Simple Strategies that Work

Management begins with your identification of your stress. It goes without saying that your inability to identify or acknowledge your stress, makes it impossible to manage or control it.

Equally important in this equation is your ability to accept those things that you can not control. Many people shape the totality of their daily conversations around things that are beyond their control. There are two clichés that come to mind here. The one that relates here is, "You are what you think about."

In other words, if your discussion of those things that are out of your control represent a source of your stress and frustration, you are doing yourself a disservice by continuing to plant seeds of discourse in your psyche.

It is imperative that you understand that your mind and body are one. If you adversely impact one you impact the other. So, your quest for healthy living and greater quality of life depends on you taking care of both.

- Make time for yourself and allow yourself to become engulfed in something that you truly enjoy. Whether it's a long walk, gardening, reading a book, sitting and watching the goings on on a body of water (lake, river, ocean side), playing or listening to music, or actively pursuing a hobby that is truly yours, it is important to have your time. This will help you to recharge your personal battery pack and do wonders for your health.

- Meditation is an approach that enables you to quiet your mind and re-synchronize your core existence to your body. In other words, meditation allows you to achieve harmony. At its optimum practice, 10 minutes in the morning and again in the evening will work wonders in calming your anxious soul.

- Deep breathing sessions are another approach to relaxation. Realizing the benefits of deep breathing are easy. Just think about the opposite. Your breathing patterns during stressful situations are characterized by shallow, rapid breaths. To the contrary, deep breathing is naturally calming to the mind and body. This method of relaxation is natural, simple and effective.

Learn the Skills of Relaxation

- Yoga and Tai Chi combine the benefits of deep breathing, meditation and muscle relaxation. This modality (as its called in the world of alternative medicine) is extremely beneficial. It represents an opportunity for physical stimulation (fitness) and has proven itself as effective in reducing headaches, anxiety, high blood pressure and shortness of breath.

- Massage and Aromatherapy have both been used to reduce stress and induce relaxation for both mind and body.

RESOURCES/TOOLS FOR YOU TO USE

I have found a combination of deep breathing and meditation to be of tremendous benefit to me over the last 21 months.

I understand from having talked with hundreds of people in putting this book together that for many, time is viewed as something that must be filled with the business of life. However, those who appreciate time use it to fulfill their lives.

I would suggest making time to claim back your life.

To help along that path here are a few recommendations:

Use the Power of Relaxation to Heal the Body!
Whether you are advanced or a beginner in the art of meditation, this interactive video creates an incredible opportunity for you to learn how to use the power of your mind to not only relax, but to heal your body on many levels. *For additional information and to pick up your copy click on the following link now*: http://sn.im/sakx2.

Lower Blood Pressure With 15 Minutes a Day of Pure Pleasure
The Breatheasy Program is one of the latest innovations in Natural Hypertension Treatments. The novel method used combines music with structured slow breathing. In addition to lowering blood pressure, this method also promotes deep relaxation, stress and anxiety relief, improved sleep and more. *For additional information and to pick up your copy click on the following link now:* http://sn.im/n6lke

Learn the Power of Aromatherapy
This book is generally regarded as a comprehensive guide to aromatherapy. The intent of the information is help you relax, work smarter and feel better. *For additional information and to pick up your copy click on the following link now:* http://sn.im/n6lr4

Learn the Skills of Relaxation

Panic Away-End Anxiety and Panic Attacks

Because I know that there are many people who suffer anxiety and panic attacks, I included this program. If this is your malady, the strong suggestion is for you to get proper medical attention. However, to bolster your options of having an effective way to relieve yourself of this situation, you may want to try this program. _For additional information and to pick up your copy click on the following link now:_ http://sn.im/n6lge

Tip No. 5

Develop a Thirst for Information and Knowledge

We live in a culture that thrives on information and knowledge, yet there's a subculture that clings to the notion that knowing less and knowing nothing is cool.

My thinking is that knowledge is what's cool.

In those communities where the socio-economic make-up is middle class or less, the key to success and affluence rests in acquiring knowledge and information and using it as leverage to catapult oneself to the next levels.

There is no way around it. Everyone that you can point to as an example of someone who "got paid" transformed themselves by acquiring information and knowledge and aggressively applying it.

The good news for all who thirst for change is that there are more ways to acquire knowledge and information now than ever before.

In many cities you can sign up for mini-courses at learning annexes or learning centers.

More formal learning opportunities are available at community colleges and universities. Many universities offer after hour adult learning academies where courses and curriculums are offered (many at reduced rates).

Then there are the online opportunities where you can even obtain advanced degrees right in the comfort of your own home.

Outside of the formal educational opportunities, there are countless ways to enrich your life with knowledge and information.

Books on any and every imaginable subject matter have been written and are available online and in bookstores.

Maybe you have specialized knowledge in an area that the world is thirsting for. Write that book and enrich the world in that way.

But in the meantime, your appetite for learning and knowledge can be fed. For those who claim to have limited time and rather not spend their free time sitting and reading, audio books can be played on your IPOD or in your car. For those of you who enjoy books but hate carrying them around, you can download them onto an electronic device (called a Kindle) that is the size of a small notebook and carry them with you.

The point of the matter is this: Knowledge is power and this power matters.

RESOURCES/TOOLS THAT YOU CAN USE

The technology that is available today is astounding. The developments continue to hit the market at a dizzying pace. The reality though, is it's easier than ever for you to keep up with those things that truly matter. In this instance, I'm talking about you having access to information. The items in this section have everything to do with giving you access.

1. IPOD. This little device is best described as a multi-functional media warehouse in your pocket. It gives you the ability to store and play music; take, store and view photos; and create, store, and play videos. As related to your new quest for information and knowledge, this device is indispensable. For those of you who don't have the time to actually read the kind of books to supercharge your personal growth, you can download them as audio books and listen to them. Click on the link that follows and take a look at two choices. You'll find them on page two of the site. http://astore.amazon.com/gsimmshealth-20.

2. KINDLE. Once again, technology has outdone itself. There used to be a time when an avid reader needed strong muscles to carry all of the magazines and books that he/she wanted to read. Imagine lugging all of that weight around with you every time you went somewhere. Well, the Kindle Wireless Reading Device solved that problem for you. With a six inch display and its slim and lightweight body (only 10.2 ounces), you can download books, newspapers, magazines, and blogs . You can create a library of up to 1500 books and hold them in the palm of your hand. It works wirelessly using 3G technology and requires NO contracts, and NO monthly fees. An Amazon.com device, you can get it here by clicking the following link: http://astore.amazon.com/gsimmshealth-20.

Tip No. 6

If You're Motivated to Do Something, DO IT NOW!

I recently read something that I totally agree with. Published in an article that appeared in Psychology Today in August of 2003, Hara Estroff Marano wrote, "There are many ways to avoid success in life, but the most sure-fire just might be procrastination. Procrastinators sabotage themselves. They put obstacles in their own path. They actually choose paths that hurt their performance."

This is another "wow" moment. Not that this is shocking, but I couldn't have said it better myself.

Procrastination is a behavior where people will defer actions, tasks or decisions to a later time. Running parallel with procrastination is stress, guilt, loss of productivity and the creation of crisis.

I felt strongly about the inclusion of this chapter in this book because I've literally talked with hundreds of people in the course of writing this book. The gamut has included young people, baby boomers and the elderly and the common thread among all of those who have recognized the need to change and improve but have not is procrastination.

The saddest of all disappointments is to know what to do and not do it because you've delayed making the decision for usually no good reason. Even worse is the person who's delayed action that would move them to a better result (again for usually no good reason) and suffered the ultimate setback that could have been avoided.

Psychologists say that procrastination affects us all, but for those whose lives are paralyzed by this, you are suffering needlessly and robbing yourself of quality of life.

Those who study this phenomenon at length say that fear is at the core of procrastination.

Now, I am not a psychologist, but I am offering information for you to contemplate based on experience and observation. If you are among those who require professional assessment and direction, by all means seek the counsel of someone who is credentialed in this area.

That said, the fast and dirty tidbits for your consideration are simple. If fear has caused you to become paralyzed along your path, you've got to become un-stuck.

When you acknowledge being motivated to do something, don't wait for the proverbial road map that surely never follows. Just Do It...and Do It Now!!!!

If You're Motivated to Do Something: Do It Now

You've got to learn to trust your instincts. It has been my experience that this is the way I receive my divinely inspired pathways. As such, you must empower yourself to think powerfully, visualize your outcomes and begin down that path RIGHT NOW, not tomorrow.

Procrastination is a rather vicious malady. The procrastinator is usually overwhelmed with stress and pressure…is typically insecure about self worth, ability and personal goals…does not know how to relax and is often times depressed.

If, however, you're just a little thrown by your fear of failure, fear of successes, fear of being alone, fear of attachment…or whatever your fear is, most fear is unfounded when you give it a good thought. Okay, acknowledge your fear, stare it in the face, and attack the mission anyway. Things usually aren't nearly as bad as you think that they are.

RESOURCES/TOOLS THAT YOU CAN USE
There are many books and programs available to help you with your procrastination. You might even go the route of professional psychological counseling. As a start though, if you sense that you need some structure in rectifying your inability to do it now, I suggest the book, *"Do It Now"* by William J. Knaus. You can use this link (http://astore.amazon.com/qsimmshealth-20) to order your copy of this book directly from my Amazon store.

Tip No. 7

Stop Accepting Advice From Everyone Wanting To Give It

The word advice is defined as an opinion or recommendation offered as a guide for action or conduct. Everyone in life (at some point) will need the advice of someone; however, the source of the advice you get and ultimately follow is important.

This is one of those topics that will assuredly touch off a firestorm of comments, but I am of the mind that this topic is important to address because I've had the opportunity to speak with thousands of people over the last 15 years of doing business and see a distinct pattern that limits the desperate individuals who are allegedly trying to do the right things.

Whenever I think about advice, my mind usually falls on syndicated columnists Dear Abby and Ann Landers who lived lives of privilege giving what I call "unauthorized or unqualified advice" on relationships, sex, love, and romance (actually all the same in the American vernacular).

In a very decided manner, I say that the advice is unauthorized because it was given by people who simply had an opinion and no training or research to quantify their positions.

The point however is not about Dear Abby or Ann Landers. The point is about what I hear when talking to the many people who take even less qualified advice from friends, and even family with hidden or egregious agendas. Have you heard the term "dream killers"?

Perhaps you even know some who fit the term perfectly. These are people who regardless of what you say or offer up for consideration will find a way to talk you out of or disparage your thoughts about any given topic. They offer their opinion in their most persuasive and articulate but unqualified voice.

Wisdom has served me well over the years. Whenever I ponder a course of action or a thought that I hold to be important, I've learned to keep those thoughts or possible courses of action to myself for several reasons.

The first of which has everything to do with the dream killing merchants who dare not to see you realize your dreams. The second reason that I keep my thoughts to myself is as vital as the first—I only seek counsel from people who are qualified to give me advice in the area that I seek counsel.

Doesn't it make sense to seek law advice from an attorney? But even there, you have to be specific. If I need advice regarding a patent, I wouldn't seek that advice from an entertainment lawyer, right?

Advice

I fondly remember the occasion where I came to a crossroad regarding a career decision. At the time, I worked as an aerospace communications consultant (a lucrative area to work in at the time although the volatility of aerospace threatened my livelihood at least three or four times a year).

A friend of mine (an aerospace facility engineer who later became my business partner) was frustrated with the craziness of aerospace at that time and considered starting a real estate and mortgage brokerage business. Now keep in mind this was at a time when those were extremely viable industries.

Before approaching my friend about his consideration, I sought and got the counsel from people (who did not know me from the elephant in the zoo) about a number of things regarding my interest in pursuing these industries at that time. These people were more than willing to share their knowledge and experience (good and bad) with me. Long story short, I used that information to make a decision to take the plunge.

The result–I rode that wave and earned a very good living for almost 15 years as a result of accepting the good counsel that I sought.

However, I just had to see what the circle of unqualified advice givers might say about what I was considering at that time.

I was not surprised at what I heard. The smart ones in the unqualified camp were non-committal. I appreciated that. If you don't know, shut up; however, that was not the norm. Those who gave themselves far too much authority came up with 800 different reasons why I shouldn't do it and some even offered options about things and professions that I should have considered (mind you none of them endeavored to do any of what they suggested).

Are you getting the point here? This is as plain as the noses on all of our faces.

Seek counsel or advice from people qualified to give it. If you're considering a course of action or a path, talk with someone who is currently doing what you are considering. I would even seek that advice from several people in that area of specialization. I'd even go so far as to say (with emphasis) seek that advice from people who don't know you. The information tends to be pure from those sources.

When they offer you their advice or opinion, by all means, pay attention. You know when someone is being genuine with you.

Help yourself and get it right the first time. Doing so will help you to avoid unnecessary stress and aggravation of mind, body and soul.

BODY

TIP No. 8

Make Fitness a Part of Your Lifestyle

For many of us, life has gotten in the way.

In other words, we've allowed life's chores and obstacles to stop us from maintaining our health.

As young people, most of us took our health for granted and started the habit of personal self abuse. And because fitness was and continues to be sold and marketed as a cosmetic result, we are still missing the point.

Of course, the look and feel of a fit body far exceeds its unattractive counterpart. But to go a little deeper allows you to discover certain realities. According to the volumes of research conducted by many clinicians studying fitness:

- A fit body functions at a more efficient level than an unfit body;

- The person with a fit body sleeps better than the person who is not fit;

- A fit body is better equipped to handle life's stresses;

- A fit body reacts to scenarios that call for its owner to make tough decisions;

- A fit person is usually less irritable and normally is less likely to get sick.

If the five aforementioned items were all of the benefits to fitness, those alone would elevate most people's quality of life significantly.

Your fitness enables your ability to maintain or continue a quality of life that is about healthy and inspired living. The simplest suggestion here is to incorporate an activity in your life that you can do everyday and be moved to exhaustion and sweat.

Need a little help in this area, check the resource/tools box.

RESOURCES/TOOLS FOR YOU TO USE
You have literally thousands of choices that are available to you.

I would rather keep your choices simple. Most people reading this book need to get started. With that in mind, these are the recommendations that make sense and will keep you encouraged along your path to a greater level of fitness.

Make Fitness A Part of Your Lifestyle

A.   Walking is one of the easiest and most beneficial exercises that anyone can do. You only need a few items to get you started. Find a good pair of walking shoes by going to any sporting goods or athletic shoe store. What's important here is getting a comfortable shoe. Don't get caught up into making your selection based on how cute or cool the shoe appears. Comfort is everything and the result is vital--move.

There are many sources and lots of information regarding the benefits of walking. Here are just two items of interest that will allow you to shape the goals of your walking program.

--Strive for walking 10,000 steps a day

It's not necessary to do this all at once. If you have a sedentary job, break your day up and take short walks throughout the day where you get in 500 steps at a time. To measure your totals, you can buy a pedometer by clicking the link below. Just place it on your belt buckle and it will record the number of steps, distance walked, and even the calories that you've burned while doing your walking.

Use this link (http://astore.amazon.com/gsimmshealth-20) for access to information, walking shoes, and a device to record your steps throughout the day.

B.   You could join a gym. I don't particularly recommend this choice because most of you are re-entering the fitness arena and just simply need to get started. The gym environment can be intimidating. Though there are trainers available to help you along the way, I still would not recommend this as a starting place. My recommendation is to do something simple that you will enjoy doing and do regularly. The key is for you to move and sweat. You must also remember that your goal is to see steady results. It's not the goal to lose 25 pounds during your first week of activity. Your goal is for the long haul—in other words, slow and steady.

C.   For those of you who might want a little more structure and can handle a little more activity, I suggest a program that I personally use. It is a very simple program that practically anyone can do. Additionally, you can add exercises and movements to it as you become more and more fit. I call it the *fast and natural* fitness program. The cost is truly minimal—less than $20, but your benefit— tremendous. You can download a copy that includes instructions on how to perform the two simple movements that will actually stimulate the whole body by clicking on this link: http://sn.im/jqz7j

TIP No. 9

Become a Student and Advocate of Proper Nutrition

This is a tricky one. Because of the proliferation of information and information sources, everyone who has desired an audience and spotlight has opened their mouths and sharpened their pencils to say something in hopes that their voice will represent the next great nutritional fad.

Well, let's step back for a hot moment. We're not talking about dieting or restricting your nutritional intake to create an ill-conceived presence of health. I'm talking about learning how to eat in a way that sustains a healthy and inspired life—not tear it down.

The reality though, is that something must be done. As a people, we are in dire straits as it relates to our denigrated health. Obesity is at epidemic proportions in almost every age category.

It used to be a time when being overweight was the province of the aging. Not anymore. Have you looked at our children lately? Many of them are clinically obese. Ruled by the fast food giants, digital games played on computers and in front of television sets, and high sugar and fat saturated snacks, our children look like miniature helium filled balloons. The rise in child hood diabetes and high blood pressure cases is appalling.

For baby boomers, there's an alarming trend of unhealthiness as well.

There are numbers of us who have endeavored to maintain a healthy living standard; however, I recently saw a report that says that (for those of us whose parents are still living) our parents are more healthy than we are.

Wow!! (I seem to use that expression a lot).

If you care to pay any attention by just casual observation, maybe you too can do an unqualified, non-scientific, but albeit shocking quantification of that report.

Indulge me for a quick second and I'll give you something to consider.

I recently wrote an article entitled, "Killing Ourselves with the Knife, Fork and Spoon".

In it, I talked about an observation at a stage play that I attended. What follows is an excerpt from that article. After reading it, just think for a minute. Have you seen the people that I describe? Are you one of them?

Become a Student and Advocate of Proper Nutrition

"...prior to the opening act, I sat in my seat awaiting the start of the play. As people finished off their drinks in the lobby they proceeded toward their seats and the auditorium filled and became abuzz with movement, music and bodies.

What's critical here are the bodies. Considering the marketing of this play, the old school demographic (35-54 year olds according to FaceBook) was in attendance.

And as for the bodies, it would be unreasonable to expect that everyone would be in shape and appear to be the pictures of health, but I have said and will continue to say (until I see it differently) that we are killing ourselves.

Many of those in attendance were decidedly overweight, huffin' and puffin' going up the short stack of steps (five) to the next level, or from their walk from the parking garage.

Please don't get this twisted. I am in no way trying to stand in judgment of those in attendance. I'm simply making a point that we should seek help and then follow the advice that will reflect a healthier result.

Many of us have poor eating habits and make even poorer eating decisions. When coupled with genetics and age (here's where the old school demographic comes into play), many of us are walking Time bombs."

Years ago, I read research that said that cancer and various other maladies of the body were primarily the result of our diets. In other words, what we eat is killing us.

There is a lot of information out there. In the resources/tools section, my recommendation will take some of the confusion out of the mix. The approach found there is simple and based on a brand of research that has nothing to do with political posturing. I have found it to be effective. It works for me and I feel it has enough merit to suggest it for consideration.

Become a Student and Advocate of Proper Nutrition

RESOURCES/TOOLS FOR YOU TO USE

I recently purchased a copy of a book called the "Healthy Urban Kitchen Cookbook". It makes for excellent reading and offers a simple, step-by-step system for shopping, cooking, and eating the world's healthiest food. Bottom line is this--if you eat in a proper fashion, you'll lose weight if you're overweight and gain weight if you're underweight. The goal though is achieving maximum health for healthy and inspired living. If you'd like to check it out, http://sn.im/jxeuf.

You'll see this in the Healthy Urban Kitchen Cookbook, but I'm going to put it here for emphasis as well. It would be of tremendous benefit for you to take a metabolic typing exam.

Your body and your body's chemistry changes more often than you might know. Have you noticed that some foods that you once enjoyed no longer agree with you? Well, the simple exam, conducted online will put you on track and specifically identify those foods that you should consume according to your individual metabolic needs.

Log on to http://www.naturalhealthyellowpages.com/metabolic/self_test.html and find out what your body is screaming at you to give to it. Truth is for many of you struggling with weight situations, your metabolic typing results will aide you in your quest to gain or lose weight.

TIP No. 10

Eat Wholesome, Organic Plant Foods

Okay, I'm aware of the difference between the price of organic fruit and vegetables as opposed to what you can pick up at the local grocery store, but I'll offer a few suggestions to help with the cost.

Every town or city has a farmer's market. Typically, these are venues that feature local merchants, farmers, and vendors. This venue offers you the opportunity to purchase fresh produce. Make it a point to talk with and develop a relationship with these vendors. Ask about their use of pesticides and other contaminants that have an ill affect on your health. Choose to purchase your fruit and veggies from the vendors that don't poison their crops. This way you'll save money and eat in the healthiest fashion.

The benefits here are many. In most cases (and if you are American), our diets don't contain enough fruit and vegetables. According to research presented by fellow web writer, Jon Tillman at JonTillman.com, 85% of our nation's children and 60% of adults do not meet the five a day recommendations for fruits and vegetables. Furthermore, 90% of American food income is spent buying processed foods.

So, as a result of your newfound affinity for a weekly trip or two to the local farmer's market, you can up your healthy intake of fruit and vegetables and at the same time, alkalinize your body (more about this in another section) while providing the ultimate defense against sickness and disease.

TIP No. 11

Take a Metabolic Profile Test

I am not surprised if you don't know what this is or have never heard of it. I became aware of this just a couple of years ago when, by virtue of experiencing bad radio reception in an area that I traveled through and being forced to listen to a talk radio program, I was exposed to metabolic typing.

So, the quick and easy answer is this. Metabolic typing is a test that's comprised of a battery of questions that when answered will classify you in a category that better determines the specific foods that you should eat based on your physiological reaction to specific food types.

Now I'm sure that this sounds like hocus pocus to those who are uninitiated; however, if you have ever wondered why some food makes you feel a certain way, or better yet, why is it that one person can eat a certain food and have no reaction and another person will eat that same meal and have a bloated feeling. You are half way there to understanding the value of a metabolic typing profile.

I recently took one such test. If for no other reason than to be able to tell you exactly how to get the best result from your pursuit of this knowledge about yourself, I paid for the test, but I will share a resource with you where you can take this test at no cost and receive the recommended food matrix that tells you what you should eat based on your typing results (which by the way are instant once you've answered all of the questions).

You can take this profile online (REMEMBER: THERE IS NO CHARGE).

Go to http://www.naturalhealthyellowpages.com/metabolic/self_test.html
Here you can take the free test online. I found it to be accurate as it rendered the same result as the test that I paid $40 for. At the end of the test, you will find out your metabolic profile and will learn the foods that you should and should not eat in order to maximize your health and wellness. The result will even make recommendations as to what supplements you should consider taking.

TIP No. 12

Change Your Drinking Water, Change Your Life

As I write this, I can not express strongly enough that drinking the right water is the number one thing that you can do to change your life for the better.

"Wow!" you say.

Naturally, the next questions are, "What are you talking about?"..."What do you mean—'the right water'?"...and the inevitable statement..."I drink *'so and so'* water. I know it's good."

The proper retort to the questions and statement above comes down to the science of your water. Considering that there is more science than we have time and space for, I'll simplify this discussion with a big picture explanation.

Without knowing the specifics about the water that you consumed when you took your last sip, if you are like 10 out of 10 people randomly sampled, you are drinking water that is acidic.

In the simplest form, the term "acidic" has to do with the measurement of your water's acidity or alkalinity on the pH (potential of hydrogen) scale. The range of the pH scale is from zero to 14 with seven being neutral.

Research has associated low pH or being acidic to disease. The same volumes of research indicate that individuals whose pH is slightly alkaline (7.2 to 7.6) have a living and sustainable body. That condition (an alkaline body) enables optimum health and is your greatest defense against the degenerative diseases that most have associated with aging (cancer, arthritis, diabetes, osteoporosis, high blood pressure, and other degenerative diseases).

Research, largely pioneered in Japan, has concluded that the easiest way to alkalinize your body is to consume hydrogen rich alkaline water.

The Water Institute of Japan continues to sit at the cutting edge of the advances made and recommended in this area. In fact, the consumption of alkaline water is common place in Japan and has been associated with the relative healthiness of the Japanese.

Considering that our bodies are 70% water, it makes sense to hydrate your body with water that supports the optimum condition of alkalinity.

Dr. Hidemitsu Hayashi, Heart Specialist and Director of the Water Institute of Japan, is one of the world's foremost authorities in this research. It was his research that essentially pioneered the development of the ionized water machines that are now common place in Japan and currently catching on here in the United States.

While many were satisfied to conclude that the alkalinity of water, by itself, was sufficient to move one's body from acidic to alkalinity, Dr. Hayashi's continued research uncovered what was to become an even greater discovery.

Dr. Hayashi discussed what he called the "hydrogen richness" of the water developed by the machines being used and marketed. He said that the hydrogen rich state was as important as the alkalinity.

His current theory now represents the summation of his many years of research and practical application of his findings which says that *drinking hydrogen rich alkaline water and consuming alkaline rich foods is the easiest and best way for mankind to avoid illness.*

He describes illness as a state where acid waste has accumulated in the body at a substantial enough rate to create the environment where the resulting illnesses can breed, dwell, and deplete our bodies of its life source. Something as simple as smelly stools can indicate just how toxic or acidic your body is.

While a good diet that is rich in antioxidants like vitamins C and E and beta-carotenes constitutes good medicine, he states that the best source of antioxidant protection against an acidic environment is water—hydrogen rich, alkaline water. Plain speak of the scientific explanations says that hydrogen rich, alkaline rich water has a low molecule weight and acts faster on all of the body's systems than any other potential substance.

SO, HOW WILL DRINKING HYDROGEN RICH ALKALINE WATER BENEFIT ME?

Many of the claims made by people who drink hydrogen rich alkaline water are nothing short of miraculous.

The positive impacts include:

--Creating more mental clarity and increased energy (due to the higher oxygenized levels of the water);

--Serving as the ultimate antioxidant. (Hydrogen rich, alkaline water attacks free radicals in the body and thus is a powerful antioxidant that is quickly assimilated in the body);

Change Your Drinking Water, Change Your Life

--Helping to balance the body's pH levels;

--Promoting weight loss. (The quick explanation is that drinking hydrogen rich, alkaline water flushes out acid waste. In doing so, the fat cells that form clusters to protect your body against acid wastes are no longer needed to protect you against the acid and thereby are eliminated as well. The result is weight loss.);

--Providing complete hydration, natural detoxification, and better body function;

--Facilitating better absorption of the nutrients from the foods you eat. (The idea here is that when you cook with hydrogen rich alkaline water, the properties of the water translate to the food making it more bio-available.);

--Better eliminatory health. (It has been noted by the medical community that greater consumption of water reduces constipation. Among the many contributors to that condition, Dr. Hayashi talks about the condition symbolized by offensive stools.);

In a published report that discusses his research (A Lecture on Water that Prevents and Cures Disease), Dr. Hayashi calls offensive stools "decay". He says that abnormal fermentation has taken place and points to the following as being the culprits:

--Hydrogen Sulfide: A strongly toxic substance with a distinctive rotten-egg odor;
--Ammonia: A strongly toxic substance with a distinctive irritating odor commonly found in public toilets;
--Histamine: A substance that triggers allergic conditions;
--Indole: A toxic, carcinogenic substance with a smell like rotten onions;
--Phenol: Recognized to be a carcinogen due to carbolic acid; and
--Nitrosamine: Known as a first-class carcinogen.

SO, HOW CAN I GET HYDROGEN RICH ALKALINE WATER TO DRINK?

Obviously, you have to reverse your current path, but the answer is remarkably easy.

In the paragraphs that follow, I am going to share the procedure that I use to make clean, great tasting water that is good for the body and promotes great health and wellness.

First and foremost, bottled water **is not the answer!!!!!!** There are numerous problems with bottled water. I'll identify them in an article on my website: GSimms-HealthandWellness.com.

Change Your Drinking Water, Change Your Life

The process for great hydrogen rich, alkaline water begins here and involves three steps.
1. Purify your water
2. Energize your water
3. Make your water Hydrogen and Alkaline Rich

The reality is that we live in a world that is supercharged on chemicals and toxins that are the hallmark of the so-called modern advances that create the lifestyle that we so love. But in the midst of lifestyle and modern advances, if we take a quick look at our drinking water, 'shock' is not a suitable description of what we're dealing with.

According to noted Alternative Health Information writer/publisher, Jon Barron, who in his book "Lessons from the Miracle Doctors", cites that drinking water in the U.S. currently contains more than 2,100 toxic chemicals known to cause cancer, cell mutation and nervous disorders.

With the introduction of some 1,000 new chemicals annually to the 100,000 that are currently in everyday uses, it is no surprise that, according to the Environmental Protection Agency (EPA), US industries generate some 79 million pounds of toxic waste each year that is not properly disposed of.

Adding insult to injury, the EPA says that our drinking water is polluted with feces, radiation and other contaminants that include the parasite cryptosporidium.

Fortunately, there's an easy way to rectify the problems associated with our drinking water. There are several purification units sold on the open market at varying prices; however I recommend the unit sold by Aquasana. Rated as the number one water filtration system in America, the Aquasana units are manufactured by Sun Water Systems, Inc. just outside of Dallas, TX. The company has been in the water filtration business for 15 years and has some 17 patents.

The unit that I use is the countertop filtration unit (**Model No. AQ-4000**). It installs in minutes to your tap water faucet (kitchen sink) and comes with a 100% guarantee for satisfaction.

The unit retails for $124.99 but you can use this link (http://snurl.com/igpvv) to purchase this unit for **$99.00**.

Additionally, you should buy a unit to attach to your showerhead. Doing so will eliminate chlorine from your shower water and stop chlorine from entering your body through your pores. (Chlorine is used as a purification agent. When ingested in liquid form, it leads to several types of cancer. Dermal absorption causes severe skin irritations).

Change Your Drinking Water, Change Your Life

The two units sold are the **AQ-4100 Shower Filtration System** which sells for $84.95—available through this link (http://snurl.com/igpvv) for **$67.99**; and the **AQ-4105 Shower Filter with Handheld Massager** which sells for $104.95 and is available through this link (http://snurl.com.igpvv) for **$83.96.**

In addition to your avoiding exposure to chlorine in your system, you will experience the side benefit of softer skin and hair in as short a time span as one week of use.

STEP 2

This step involves a process that I was just recently introduced to.

Substances (in this case water) are measured for their energy by the Bovis Scale (named after the French physicist who developed it). Living organisms have as their reference point an amount of 6,500 bovis. Anything below 6,500 bovis is considered in negative range or life-detracting. A measurement above 6,500 is considered positive energy or life enhancing. The desired range for humans is between 8,000 and 10,000 bovis.

With the average measurement of tap water registering at 3,000 – 4,000 bovis, the energy of the water needs to be raised so that it can render its optimal utilization for your body.

Raising the bovis level of your water is accomplished by reversing the spin of the atoms. The simplest way to accomplish this is via the use of a product developed by a group of German scientists.

You simply pour your water into an energy mug or pitcher and within minutes the science of the mug/pitcher changes the direction of the atoms and thereby raises the bovis or energy level of your water.

You can use this link (Click here) to purchase either a mug (treats 17.5 oz at a time) or a pitcher (treats 48 oz.). The **Mug** sells for **$34.95** and the **Pitcher** sells for **$74.95**.

STEP THREE – Make Your Water Hydrogen and Alkaline Rich

This is where the rubber meets the road. The process is remarkably simple and involves a product that only costs $79.95 and lasts for some six months.

Developed by Dr. Hayashi, this product does not depend on expensive machines that cost anywhere from $700 to $4,000. Neither does this product depend on chemical droplets that are added to your water (haven't you suffered enough from chemical contamination?).

Change Your Drinking Water, Change Your Life

His product was originally known as the Hydrogen Producing Water Stick.

The stick is actually composed of a very important mineral—Magnesium.

You simply place this in your purified/energized water and presto—you have created hydrogen rich, alkaline water.

Recommendation: I store my purified water in an air tight glass container that holds 68 oz. I do not refrigerate this water. I place two hydrogen-rich water sticks in that container and fill it with purified water from my Aquasana AQ-4000 unit. When I am ready to drink some of this water, I fill my bovis raising mug and let it sit for at least three minutes before consuming. Over the course of the day, I consume roughly half of my bodyweight in ounces.

The result is good tasting, healthy water.

You can get your hydrogen-rich water stick through this link (http://snurl.com/igrrx). When placing your order, use the friend code number (2110).

RESOURCES/TOOLS FOR YOU TO USE

Over the last several months, I've had an opportunity to test, experiment and actually discover the merits of hydrogen-rich alkaline water and can attest to the difference it has made for me. Prior to this, water was something that I took for granted. The consensus was that if the water was said to be clean, then it was good. The reality however, is that the consensus is wrong. The information to prove the consensus being wrong is readily available and only took a little research. This report reflects the collective research that I did. As a result, I've made decisions that proved beneficial to my health by following the simple steps featured in this chapter. It would be wise, helpful and healthy for you too.

Originally, this chapter was written for another of my publications. Considering that the format was slightly different, you will note that the resources/tools are actually present-ed within the chapter as links. Please go back and click on the various links for access to the products discussed.

TIP No. 13

Caution: Do Not Put That Toothpaste in Your Mouth

Let's start with the proverbial million dollar questions.

What brand of toothpaste is your favorite? How did that brand become your favorite? Was it a traditional choice? Was it taste? Was it their marketing? Did they have one of your favorite commercials? Do you choose your toothpaste on the basis of price?

Like many other things that we do on a daily basis, the above questions and subsequent choices seem insignificant and are very much taken for granted, right?

Well, try this fact on for size. The average tube of toothpaste has some 16 different chemicals in it that for the most part are injurious to your health.

Some create mild impacts on your health while others create such grave health consequences, it's a true wonder that they're allowed on the market.

Truth is, a little research and knowledge from sources like www.sci-toys.com, www.wikipedia.com, www.cosmeticdatabase.com will reveal that the 16 or 17 chemicals have some 300-400 different aliases. So, regardless as to how they're masked on product labels, the recommendation is **DON'T PUT THAT TOOTH PASTE IN YOUR MOUTH**—unless of course, you don't care about the erosion of your health and the eventual loss of your teeth.

In all fairness, I'll attempt to present an abbreviated version of the highlights of the research that I did.

I'll start by presenting the common listings of the varied chemicals. I'll tell you why they're part of the ingredient list, highlight some side effects and provide other tidbits of information that I feel are of importance.

Generally speaking, as a people, we have to get back to common sense consumption. A naturopathic doctor that I know perhaps said it best when I heard him admonish someone by saying this, *"If you can't pronounce the ingredients, don't put it in your mouth."*

Stannous Fluoride
Known also as TIN DIFLUORIDE; TIN FLUORIDE; TIN FLUORIDE (SNF2)

This ingredient is described as a white crystal substance designed to protect teeth enamel from bacteria or cavities.

Do Not Put That Toothpaste in Your Mouth

Side Effects include: Stains teeth, causes pitting, brown spots and uneven striped enamel. In extreme cases, this substance can cause allergic reactions including rash, itching/swelling of the face/tongue/throat, dizziness and breathing complications. The substance is also known to cause cancer.

Cosmeticdatabase.com rates this substance as a moderate hazard at a 6 on a scale from 0 – 10.

Sodium Fluoride
Known also as SODIUM FLUORIDE (NAF)

Sodium Fluoride is described as a white crystal substance designed to protect teeth enamel from bacteria or cavities.

Side Effects include: Stains teeth, causes pitting, brown spots and uneven striped enamel. In extreme cases, this substance can cause allergic reactions including rash, itching/swelling of the face/tongue/throat, dizziness and breathing complications. The substance is also known to cause cancer, reproductive problems and can linger in human and wildlife tissue for years. The substance is known to cause mouth and gum irritation.

Cosmeticdatabase.com rates this substance as a high hazard at a 9 on a scale from 0 – 10.

Sodium Monofluorophosphate
Known also as MFP; PHOSPHOROFLUORIDIC ACID, SODIUM SALT; SODIUM PHOSPHOROFLUORIDATE; SODIUM SALT PHOSPHOROFLUORIDIC ACID

Sodium Monofluorophosphate is described as a white crystal substance designed to protect teeth enamel from bacteria or cavities.

Side Effects: This substance is known to cause cancer and is linked to developmental and reproductive toxicity, infertility and birth defects. The substance is also known to have a negative impact on the nervous system.

Cosmeticdatabase.com rates this substance as a moderate hazard at a 6 on a scale from 0 – 10.

Do Not Put That Toothpaste in Your Mouth

Hydrated Silica

Known also as HYDROSILICIC ACID; PRECIPITATED SILICA; SILICA GEL; SILICA HYDRATE; SILICIC ACID; SILICIC ACID HYDRATE; SILICON DIOXIDE HYDRATE; HYDRATED SILICA; and SILICA GEL

Hydrated Silica is described as a transparent gel used as an abrasive substance in toothpaste. This substance is also used in hair coloring and bleaching, in sunscreens, make-up, as an exfoliant/scrub, as a cleanser, and for nail treatment.

Side Effects: This substance is known to cause cancer and is known as a bioaccumulative (which means that it resists the normal chemical breakdown and thus can linger in wildlife and human tissues for years.

Cosmeticdatabase.com rates this substance as a low hazard at a 2 on a scale from 0 – 10.

Ammonium Lauryl Sulfate

Known also as DODECYL AMMONIUM SULFATE; SULFURIC ACID, MONODODECYL ESTER, AMMONIUM SALT; AMMONIUM SALT SULFURIC ACID, MONODODECYL ESTER; MONODODECYL ESTER AMMONIUM SALT SULFURIC ACID; AMMONIUM DODECYL SULPHATE; NEOPON LAM

Ammonium Lauryl Sulfate is described as a yellow, viscous liquid. It's an anionic surfactant which means that it is a wetting agent used to make a liquid wetter. Its use in toothpaste is as a foaming agent and detergent. This substance is also used in shampoos, as a bodywash, hair coloring and bleaching, as a facial cleaner, a conditioner, in dandruff/scalp treatments, in liquid hand soaps, in acne treatments, as an exfoliant/scrub, and as a hair relaxer.

Side Effects: This substance is known to cause irritations in oral membranes and is used under strict industrial and governmental guidelines. The toxicity impacts the cardiovascular system, can cause cancer and is known as a bioaccumulative (which means that it resists the normal chemical breakdown and thus can linger in wildlife and human tissues for years.

Cosmeticdatabase.com rates this substance as a low hazard at a 2 on a scale from 0 – 10.

Do Not Put That Toothpaste in Your Mouth

Lauryl Sarcosinate
Known also as GLYCINE, NDODECYLNMETHYL, SODIUM SALT; SODIUM N-DODECYL-N-METHYLGLYCINATE

Lauryl Sarcosinate is actually a replacement for the family of sulfates normally used in the manufacture of toothpaste. It too is described as a yellow, viscous liquid. However, this substance is an amino acid and is milder on the skin and oral membranes and can be used without causing irritation to the skin and gums. Its use in toothpaste is as a foaming agent and detergent.. This substance is also used in shampoos, as a bodywash, as a facial cleanser, in cosmetic foundations, in tooth whiteners, and as an exfoliant/scrub.

Side Effects: This substance is known to cause cancer. It is linked to toxicity impacts of the cardiovascular system, digestive system, and respiratory system. It is linked also to toxicity of wildlife, fish, and plant life.

Cosmeticdatabase.com rates this substance as a low hazard at a 1 on a scale from 0 – 10.

Allantoin
Known also as (2,5-DIOXO-4-IMIDAZOLIDINYL) UREA; GLYOXYLDIUREID; GLYOXYLDIUREIDE; GLYOXYLIC DIUREIDE; UREA, 5-UREIDOHYDAN-TOIN; (2,5-DIOXO-4-IMIDAZOLIDINYL) - UREA; UREA, (2,5DIOXO4IMIDAZOLIDINYL)

Allantoin is a white, odorless, tasteless crystal or powder used to relieve skin irritation caused by soaps, detergents, acids and alkalies found primarily in skin care products. Allantoin is commonly known as an agent to promote wound healing and tissue formation.

This substance can also be found in: facial moisturizers, anti-aging products, facial cleansers, sunscreen products, eye creams, lipstick, acne treatments, after shave products and facial masks.

Side Effects: There are no known determinable risks to this substance as of this writing.

Cosmeticdatabase.com rates this substance as a low hazard at a 0 on a scale from 0 – 10.

Tetrasodium Pyrophosphate
Known also as ANHYDROUS SODIUM PYROPHOSPHATE; DIPHOSPHORIC AC-ID, TETRASODIUM SALT; SODIUM POLYPHOSPHATE; SODIUM PYROPHOS-PHATE; TSPP; TETRASODIUM SALT DIPHOSPHORIC ACID

Do Not Put That Toothpaste in Your Mouth

Tetrasodium Pyrophosphate is described as a pH buffer. In toothpaste, this substance is used to remove calcium and magnesium from saliva. The benefit is to allegedly remove the potential of build up of damaging plaque and tarter from the teeth. In other products, this substance is used as a dough binder/conditioner in soy based meat alternatives; as a thickening agent in instant puddings, and as a water softener in detergents.

Side Effects: This substance is known as a bioaccumulative (which means that it resists normal chemical breakdown and thus can linger in wildlife and human tissues for years.) Additionally, the substance is linked to toxicity of the following biological systems: cardiovascular, stomach and digestive, and respiratory.

Cosmeticdatabase.com rates this substance as a low hazard at a 2 on a scale from 0 – 10.

Acrylic

Known also as (PMMA, PLEXIGLASS, METHACRYLATE COPOLYMER, OCTYLACRYLAMIDE/ACRYLATES/BUTYLAMINOETHYL

This substance is more likely to be listed among ingredients as ACRYLIC POLYMER. While research data did not explain its use in toothpaste, it is commonly used by manufacturers in their products.

This substance can also be found in: tooth whiteners, baby lotion, vapor rubs, nail glue, and nail polish.

Side Effects: There are no known determinable risks to this substance as of this writing.

Cosmeticdatabase.com rates this substance as a low hazard at a 0 on a scale from 0 – 10.

Polyethylene Glycol

Known also as PEG-n, PEG-6, PEG-7, etc.

Polyethylene Glycol is in the family of a long chain of polymers. It's a thickening agent and used in toothpaste for tartar control. This substance is also used in oral pain relief products, as a lubricant/spermicide, in styling gels and lotions, for pain relief, in anti-itch/rash creams, in facial cleansers, mascara, in anti-fungal treatments and body oils.

Side Effects include: The substance is known to cause cancer, reproductive problems (to include birth defects) and is suspected to be contaminated with other highly toxic impurities (such as ethylene oxide and 1.4-dioxane). As a bioaccumulative, it resists normal chemical breakdown in the environment and can linger in human and wildlife tissue for years. The substance is linked to toxicity of the following biological systems: cardiovascular, stomach and digestive, and respiratory. The substance is also known to be found as a contaminant of water and food products. This substance causes disruption to the natural function of the endocrine system and does irritate the skin, eyes and lungs.

Cosmeticdatabase.com rates this substance as a high hazard at 7–10 on a scale from 0–10.

Polyproylene Glycol
Known also as HEXAETHYLENE GLYCOL; POLYETHYLENE GLYCOL 300

Polyproylene Glycol is in the family of a long chain of polymers. It's a thickening agent and used in toothpaste for tartar control. This substance is also used as a solvent. The substance can also be found in tooth whiteners, facial cleansers, anti-aging products, facial moisturizers, eye makeup removers, makeup foundation, body sprays, and body washes.

Side Effects include: The substance requires strict regulation for its use and is suspected to be contaminated with other highly toxic impurities (such as ethylene oxide and 1.4-dioxane). The substance is linked to toxicity of the following biological systems: cardiovascular, stomach and digestive, and respiratory. This substance is also linked to being toxic and damaging to the human nervous system.

Cosmeticdatabase.com rates this substance as a medium to high hazard at 4 – 7 on a scale from 0 – 10.

Sodium Carbonate Peroxide
Known also as CARBONIC ACID, DISODIUM SALT, COMPD. WITH HYDROGEN PEROXIDE; PEROXY SODIUM CARBONATE; SODIUM PERCARBONATE; COMPD. WITH HYDROGEN PEROXIDE CARBONIC ACID, DISODIUM SALT; DISODIUM SALT COMPD. WITH HYDROGEN PEROXIDE CARBONIC ACID; CARBONIC ACID DISODIUM SALT, COMPD. WITH HYDROGEN PEROXIDE (H2O2) (2:3) ; DISODIUM CARBONATE, COMPOUND WITH HYDROGEN PER-OXIDE (2:3) ; DISODIUM CARBONATE, HYDROGEN PEROXIDE (2:3)

This substance is described as a white granule that breaks down sodium carbonate and hydrogen peroxide. It acts as a bleach and anti-microbial agent.

The substance can also be found in tooth whiteners and mouthwash.

Do Not Put That Toothpaste in Your Mouth

Side Effects include: As a bioaccumulative, it resists normal chemical breakdown in the environment and can linger in human and wildlife tissue for years. This substance is also linked to being toxic and damaging to the human nervous system. The substance is also linked to toxicity of the following biological systems: cardiovascular, stomach and digestive, and respiratory.

Cosmeticdatabase.com rates this substance as a low hazard at 2 on a scale from 0 – 10.

Sodium Saccharin
Known also as 1,2-BENZISOTHIAZOL-3 (2H) -ONE, 1,1-DIOXIDE, SODIUM SALT, DIHYDRATE; O-BENZOYLSULFIMIDE SODIUM SALT; CRYSTAL-LOSE; 1,1-DIOXIDE-1,2-BENZISOTHIAZOL-3 (2H) -ONE, SODIUM SALT, DIHY-DRATE; SACCHARINE, SODIUM SALT; SACCHARIN SODIUM; SODUIM SACCHARINE; DIHYDRATE

This substance is a colorless, odorless, sweet tasting white powder used as a low calorie sweetner.

The substance can also be found in tooth whiteners, mouthwash, lip gloss, lip plumper, oral pain relief, lip balm, lipstick, and breath fresheners.

Side Effects include: This substance is known to cause cancer and reproductive disorders that include infertility and birth defects. This substance is known to disrupt the function of the endocrine system. This substance is also linked to being toxic and damaging to the human nervous system. The substance is also linked to toxicity of the following biological systems: cardiovascular, stomach and digestive, and respiratory.

Cosmeticdatabase.com rates this substance as a low hazard at 2 on a scale from 0 – 10.

Triclosan
Known also as 5-CHLORO-2- (2,4-DICHLOROPHENOXY) PHENOL; PHENOL, 5-CHLORO-2- (2,4-DICHLOROPHENOXY) -; 2,4,4'-TRICHLORO-2'-HYDROXY DIPHENYL ETHER.

This substance is described as a white powder and used as an antibacterial and antifungal agent. Related to hexachlorophene, it kills germs by interfering with the enzymes necessary for fatty-acid synthesis.

The substance can also be found in deodorants, liquid hand soaps, facial cleansers, acne treatments, body washes, moisturizers, body sprays and lipsticks.

Do Not Put That Toothpaste in Your Mouth

<u>Side Effects include</u>: This substance is known to cause cancer and reproductive disorders that include infertility and birth defects. The substance requires strict regulation for its use and is suspected to be contaminated with other highly toxic impurities (such as chloroform and dioxin). As a bioaccumulative, it resists normal chemical breakdown in the environment and can linger in human and wildlife tissue for years. This substance is a known irritant to the skin, eyes and lungs. This substance is known to disrupt the function of the endocrine system. The substance is linked to toxicity of the following biological systems: cardiovascular, stomach and digestive, and respiratory. Additionally, this substance is toxic to wildlife to include fish, plant life and other wild organisms.

Cosmeticdatabase.com rates this substance as a high hazard at 8 on a scale from 0 – 10.

Hexachlorophene
Known also as BIS (3,5,6-TRICHLORO-2-HYDROXYPHENYL) -METHANE; 2,2'-DIHYDROXY-3,3',5,5'6,6'-HEXACHLORODIPHENYLMETHANE; HEXACHLO-ROFEN; 3,3',4,4',6,6'-HEXACHLORO-2,2'-METHYLENEDIPHENOL; HEXACHLO-ROPHEN; 2,2'-METHYLENEBIS (3,4,6-TRICHLOROPHENOL) ; PHENOL, 2,2' -METHYLENEBIS (3,4,6-TRICHLORO-.

This substance is related to Triclosan. It is typically used as a deodorant agent.

<u>Side Effects include</u>: This substance is known to cause cancer and reproductive disorders that include infertility and birth defects. The substance requires strict regulation for its use. As a bioaccumulative, it resists normal chemical breakdown in the environment and can linger in human and wildlife tissue for years. Requiring special precautions for its use, this substance can cause acute responses as an occupational hazard and is toxic to the human nervous system. This substance is a known irritant to the skin, eyes and lungs. This substance is known to disrupt the function of the endocrine system. The substance is linked to toxicity of the following biological systems: cardiovascular, stomach and digestive, and respiratory. Additionally, this substance is toxic to wildlife to include fish, plant life and other wild organisms.

Cosmeticdatabase.com rates this substance as a high hazard at 10 on a scale from 0 – 10.

<u>RESOURCES/TOOLS FOR YOU TO USE</u>

The natural and easy recommendation is in support of any product that is verifiable as being made from natural ingredients; however, **don't be fooled by product advertising.** In testing this theory, I went to a high end food store and picked up a handful of toothpastes and noticed a few things.

Do Not Put That Toothpaste in Your Mouth

First, the more expensive products that claimed to be natural and organic, in most cases, weren't as promoted. While they claimed to not contain preservatives and sugars as your name brand counterparts do, they all contained some of the above listed chemicals as their main ingredients. The result is that you've been made to believe that these products are safe and manufactured in a way that ensures observance of your health when in fact, that's not the case.

Your new reality is this, if you choose to feel better-beginning today—no more bleeding gums, no more sensitive lips, canker sores (caused by the chemicals in the toothpaste), and reduce the overall negative impact to your health, then here's my recommendation.

The product that helps you to get your mouth together is called Tooth Soap. You can reach them online through this link http://eCa.sh/76bu . When you get to that site, there's a special offer that you can take advantage of through the link that I gave you. That offer includes one of several flavors of Tooth Soap plus a booklet entitled, "The Perfect Prescription For Your Teeth".

If you can afford the price of this offer, it is well worth the money because it gives more detailed information about the product as well as additional details about their natural approach to taking great care of your teeth. If I can use the proverbial "trust me" here, then trust me on this one. This information will save you thousands of dollars at the dentist and work wonders at protecting, preserving, and restoring your health. After all, your mouth is a major gateway for everything that involves your health.

The shop online portion of the site presents other offers as well.

TIP No. 14

Eat 4-5 Meals A Day

This chapter should perhaps have a new title. For the record, it should properly be entitled, "Re-Program Your Metabolism with 4-5 Small Meals a Day".

I'm making this point from the outset because, for many of the people reading this book, the goal is to glean from it information that will tilt the scales of health back toward an enriched, wholesome life.

That means that you're needing to lose pounds of unnecessary fat that have done nothing more than made you ill.

So, this tip is one that can quickly put you in the direction of reclaiming your health.

The Basics and the Problem

If you are like most people, you think that losing weight is a result of eating fewer meals, restricting calories, and restricting food choices.

Furthermore, the average person will look at the scale, see that they may have dropped a few pounds, and feel wholeheartedly that their plan is working...at least until, they've checked the scale two weeks later to discover that not only is their plan not working, they've gained weight.

So what happened?

Their body has gone into starvation mode.

Instead of shedding the unwanted pounds, their body has made an adjustment and decided to store all caloric intake instead. This happens because the biology of your body believes that it is not going to get food on a regular basis. As a result, its natural instinct to survive tells it that it needs to store everything being put in it because it is not getting a regular input of what it needs.

Now, in your distress, you decide to starve it further (you become more diligent about starving yourself), you may eventually lose some weight but you'll feel awful, have little or no energy, suffer extreme bouts of mood swings and slow your metabolism even further.

The Answer Is

While this may not make sense to you, it works...and science proves it does.

Eat 4-5 Meals a Day

Eat several well rounded meals each day and watch the magic of the science that governs your body. The goal would be to eat something every two to three hours. What you eat is important. Check out tip number 11 (metabolic typing). When you combine knowing what you (specifically you) should eat with eating four to five small meals each day, your new fat burning metabolism will incinerate the fat that you're carrying and return you to the land of healthy.

Your Benefits Are

You will gain a new super-charged metabolism that burns fat rather than store it. As a result, your body will burn more calories (even when you are at rest). You will also notice that you'll have more energy.

Another benefit of this kind of nutritional consumption plan (let's ditch the word diet) is that your blood sugar levels will stabilize. There are huge benefits here that have everything to do with your cravings. In other words, when your blood sugar levels are spiking, you crave nutrients. Usually, you'll satisfy these cravings by snacking on junk food. When you eat junk, you suffer the fate of needing the information in this article.

Another benefit to you is that your body will function at a higher rate of efficiency. It will promote better digestion and utilization of the nutrients found in the food.

A benefit that is very important to your weight loss effort is the conservation of muscle tissue. Did you know that when you starve yourself (and consequently go into starvation mode) your body will burn anything available (including muscle). When your body burns muscle for fuel, it slows down your metabolism and promotes the storage of fat.

I would be remiss in not taking some time to discuss your fluid intake at this point. Not discussing it could sabotage your efforts.

From the hundreds of people that I talked with while writing this book, it is evident that, many people pay little attention to the fluids that are consumed. From the coffee to the sugary fruit juices, from the colas and other pops to the energy drinks, from the beers to the wine, we can easily douse the effects of good nutritional consumption with ill advised fluid consumption.

Some estimates, based on research and information published from various sources, find that 75% of Americans are chronically dehydrated.

For years, you've heard that you should drink eight eight-ounce glasses of water a day for good health. However, most health and fitness people will tell you that you should consume one-half ounce of good alkaline water (see Tip No. 12) for every pound that you weigh. In other words, if you weigh 240 pounds, you should spread the consumption of 120 ounces of water over your day. Equally important is when you drink your water or anything else.

We've grown accustomed to having a beverage with our meals. When we do that, however, we create digestive problems.

The digestive enzymes that break down your food are compromised when you wash your food down with a beverage. The result is that the food that you eat will sit in your stomach much longer and ultimately require more energy and involvement from your body to process. The bottom line is…that is not very efficient and will contribute to your being overweight or ill.

My suggestion is that you drink your water before eating and at least one hour after eating (if you must consume beverages after your meal).

RESOURCES/TOOLS FOR YOU TO USE

I am convinced of the importance of getting a handle on your food consumption. The problem that I've discovered from talking to so many people is that very few of us ever consider that our eating plan should be tailor made for us (individually).

To help you find out the specific foods that work for you (individually), I strongly suggest that you take a **metabolic typing test**. In a matter of minutes, you can find out what you should eat and why. You can get this information online at no cost to you (free) by clicking on the link that follows:
http://www.naturalhealthyellowpages.com/metabolic/self_test.html

Once you have the results from your metabolic typing test, it would be a good idea to pick up a copy of the "Healthy Urban Kitchen Cookbook".

Not only does it make for good reading, it offers a simple, step-by-step system for shopping, cooking and eating the world's healthiest food.

Here is a good place for me to add that you should also prepare as many as (hopefully all) of your meals at home. The benefit is simple. When you prepare your food, you know what's in it. You control the ingredients (salt, fat, etc.). Understanding that, you should avoid fast food restaurants as much as possible. They are not the place to frequent if your desire is healthy eating.

To pick up your copy of the "Healthy Urban Kitchen Cookbook", click this link now:
http://sn.im/jxeuf

Tip No. 15

Eat Grass Fed Beef, Free Range Chickens and Wild Fish

The doom and gloom merchants that have created the most wide-spread obesity and the greatest reliance on prescription drugs in the history of our nation have grossly misled masses of people by peddling fear and bad information. The promotion of greater consumption of grain products and the ever popular suggestion to avoid red meat is at the center of the buzz and the problems.

Hopefully this section can provide some much needed accurate information to help you in your quest toward optimum nutrition.

In making my point about being misled with bad information, a very good friend of mine told me that his son sent him an email that extolled the virtues of avoidance of meat because of recent research that concluded that such consumption was linked to a greater incidence of cancer.

Considering that the research was covered as a news story and was aired on television and seen in print, his response was in line with most people who saw or read the same or similar coverage.

He told me that he would cut back on red meat because he did want to be proactive and observe good preventative measures.

I responded by giving him a more accurate account of what he should use to make a decision regarding his red meat consumption.

THE PROBLEM

The problem is not with red meat in general. The problem is with what red meat you're talking about.

Unfortunately, the majority of the U.S. population eats meat (beef and chicken) that was raised on commercial factory farms.

The livestock and chickens raised on those farms are fed grain and a battery of hormones and stimulants to fatten them quickly. It's very simple...the sooner they can reach marketable weight, the sooner they get to market and your table. That translates to dollars in the pockets of everyone along that path.

In the process though, your health suffers because grain feed depletes vital nutrients from the meat that lands on your table. Additionally, you will ingest greater amounts of the hormones and stimulants that were given to those cows or chickens.

Eat Grass Fed Beef, Chicken and Wild Fish

The factory farmed, grain fed, hormone injected beef and chicken that you buy from your grocery store has significantly higher percentages of fat and virtually no omega-3 fatty acids. So, yes, if this is what your diet consists of, and most Americans eat huge amounts of this kind of meat, then yes, you're a candidate for cancer.

ADDITIONAL INFORMATION

The Food and Drug Administration recommends eating grains as the predominant food that one should ingest, but most people actually do well to avoid grains altogether. Long story short, rice and flour wreaks havoc on most bodies.

Do you remember how, as a child, you made glue—perhaps as a science project—using those two food stuffs?

Generally speaking, that experiment was poignant and is of interest here. Eating those products, for the most part, makes glue internally. Our system then carries this glue throughout the body and pastes this along the walls of our arteries and of course we all know that this is not a good thing, right?

Even considering the benefits of their fiber content, better choices for fiber are fruit and vegetables.

THE RESOLUTION OF THE PROBLEM.

The answer is GRASS FED BEEF AND GRASS FED-FREE RANGE CHICKENS.

There are tremendous benefits gained from avoiding the commercially produced meat and buying the grass fed alternative.

The highlights are as follows:
- Grass fed beef and chicken are lower in fat than their grain fed counterparts. By comparison a grass fed sirloin steak has about one-half to one-third less fat than its commercially grown grain fed counterpart.
- Grass fed beef has about the same amount of fat as skinless chicken and will actually contribute to lowering your LDL cholesterol levels.
- Since grass fed beef is lower in calories, if the typical consumption was changed to the grass fed variety, the average American would save 17,733 calories a year. If nothing else in the diet changed, that person would lose 6 pounds a year.
- Eating grass fed beef, while lowering fat, would raise your consumption of omega-3 fatty acids by two to six times.

Eat Grass Fed Beef, Chicken and Wild Fish

- Omega-3 fatty acids are critical to a healthy heart.
  - Lowers blood pressure
  - Regulates the heartbeat
  - Lowers the incidence of depression, schizophrenia, attention deficit disorder, Alzheimer's and cancer. Commonly found in seafood, flaxseeds and walnuts, grass fed animals are abundant in omega-3 fatty acids. It's in the grass.
- Grass Fed red meat does not produce adverse consequences to your health (if your body reacts well to meat in accordance with your metabolic type). Grass Fed meat has the proper ratio of Omega-3 and Omega-6 fatty acids that the body craves and is an even better source than Salmon.

FOR THE FISH LOVERS: FARMED VS WILD CAUGHT

It really pays to ask questions these days.

Practically everything that we do has been touched by technology and the mindset of either "more" or "more quickly".

When it comes to the seafood that is available to you, the accepted norm of fishermen on boats catching the daily offerings at your local restaurant has changed tremendously also.

The growing world population coupled with the increased demand for fish as a viable protein choice has created the fish farming industry. And as one might expect, this option, while assisting in meeting worldwide demands, faces production challenges that are addressed by the utilization of synthetic or supplemental products and methodologies not normally found in nature.

Because fish are carnivorous by nature, the feed and oils that support this system of breeding fish for market consumption are sustained by the scavenging of open-ocean fish—the practice of which destroys the natural eco-system of the ocean to support the manufactured life development on the farms.

The risks and realities of purchasing and consuming farm raised fish include: destruction of the eco-system, drug, chemical and hormonal contamination of the product, product infections, worms, bacteria and other contaminants.

NUMBERS FOR YOUR CONSIDERATION
According to the TIME Magazine article, "Fish Farming's Growing Dangers" written by Ken Stir and published on September 19, 2007 here are some numbers of note:

Eat Grass Fed Beef, Chicken and Wild Fish

- The seafood industry is estimated to produce $78 billion in sales each year and has grown by 9% each year since 1975, making it the fastest growing food group.
- For every 2.2 pounds of high-protein fishmeal fed to farmed fish, some 10 pounds of open-ocean fish are caught and used to make this feed.
- Some 37% of all global seafood being caught is now ground into feed, up from 7.7% in 1948.
- Roughly 45% of the global production of fishmeal and fish oil is used as feed to the world's livestock industry, up from 10% in 1988.

RESOURCES/TOOLS FOR YOU TO USE

I have become a stickler about my food consumption. The past 21 months have taught me to be extremely persistent about this. I maintain this level of focus as if my life depends on it…because it does.

When it comes down to local choices about buying grass fed meat, I buy from the Whole Food Store. When dealing with the butcher, ask specifically for grass fed products.

My preference though, is to buy my beef online from Gourmet Pasture Beef. Their pricing is great and their product is considered excellent by all standards. To check them out and order product from them, use the following link: http://sn.im/tbkp6

I have become even more picky when buying fish. After lots of personal research combined with the research of others, I've settled on one supplier. This supplier catches his fish in the open waters of Alaska and has consistently tested free of all contaminants (including mercury). To check out and order from Vital Choice, you may use the following link: http://sn.im/tbkqw

Tip No. 16

No Ice Please

If your schedule is like most, sometime today you were a customer at some restaurant or eatery and of course you ordered something to drink…coke, sprite, iced tea.

The natural expectation is that you'll receive nothing other than what you ordered, but did you ever consider that your favorite drink is possibly dirtier than toilet water because of the ice?

One study done in Chicago tested the ice at various restaurants and found that more than one of every five has more bacteria and fecal matter in their ice cubes than in a random testing of toilet water.

While the full details of the results indicated that the bacteria found was not necessarily dangerous to the average person, it becomes apparent that you (the consumer) must take more responsibility to protect your health.

Okay, so your reaction might be to deny this possibility in your daily experience for a variety of reasons, but seriously, your knowledge of the possibility of becoming sick or even dying as a result of having your favorite iced beverage in a public eatery might cause you to change your drinking habits or wait to chill your drinks yourself…at home.

In a report that aired on MSNBC in July of 2006, the story was told of a healthy 15-year old boy who after a round of golf at a junior golf tournament with dozens of other healthy youngsters took what became a deadly drink of cold water. The water was supposed to be refreshment for the junior golfers in the heated conditions.

His death was traced to choking on his vomit overnight as the result of gastrointestinal illness (Norovirus) caused by drinking tainted water (found in the coolers) that was available for the young golfers. Officials surmised that a sick employee who had not washed his hands contaminated the ice in the coolers.

WHILE YOU'RE SAYING NO TO ICE…
It's a good idea to also pass on the nuts, pretzels and chips that sit in opened containers at bars. All of these snack items present the same problem. They are contaminated with human waste.

Studies, similar to the ice study, have confirmed that fecal matter, E Coli, urine and associated forms of bacteria were routinely found in the aforementioned containers whenever tests were done. This should not be shocking information. All of us have been in the rest rooms of our favorite watering holes. If you pay just a little attention, you'll notice that probably less than half of the people using the facilities will actually wash their hands afterwards. Guess where those unwashed hands go once they return to their drinking buddies—that's correct…right into the bowl of chips, nuts, pretzels, candy, etc. sitting atop the bar. The suggestion then is simple. If you're not interested in ingesting their waste matter, just say no to eating out of the chips, nuts, pretzels and candies served in open containers at such establishments.

RESOURCES/TOOLS FOR YOU TO USE

Because you aren't privileged to all of the information about who's handling your food and drink (or even ice), it makes sense to consider how knowing the possibilities and observing a few rules for personal "good practices" might help you avoid having your health compromised.

It makes sense to:
--Order your drinks without ice when eating out. If you like lemon or lime in your drink, have the waiter to place them on a saucer (there are reports that state that they are potentially a source of similar contamination).
--While you won't be able to see everyone who might possibly handle your food at a restaurant, if you see that someone is sick, don't eat there.
--Make every effort to eat as many meals as possible at home. There you can control the possible contamination to your food by practicing great cleanliness.
--Do not allow your sick children to have access to food and food preparation areas. There is no such thing as children's germs and grown-up germs.
--Avoid self-service and buffet food courts and vending machines. I have person-ally witnessed some of the nastiest goings-on at those styled eateries. If you're not convinced, pay attention to people's behavior at those self-service food areas.

- I have seen people grab food with their hands--use an already used plate or container and either drip or pour a portion of what they decided that they didn't want back into the serving source;
- I've seen children play in the food at serving stations;
- I've seen people lick their hands and put them in the food at serving stations;
- I've seen people cough into the food at the serving stations;
- I've seen people sneeze into the food at the serving stations;
- I've seen people blow their noses into handkerchiefs, hold that same handkerchief over the serving area and invariably drag that handkerchief over food in the serving stations;
- I've seen people walk off streets (having dirty hands) and go directly to the serving areas and handle food;
- I've witnessed people leaving the bathroom (without washing their hands) and head to the food serving area and do all of the above.

Need anyone say anymore?

Tip No. 17

Throw Your Microwave Away

For many, the microwave oven represents technology at its finest. The thought of instant everything...from the freezer or lazy susan to the dining room table in a matter of seconds was supposed to mean that mom might have more time and that the family could actually use the saved time to have more "quality time".

Well, that's not the way things played out. Microwave ovens have contributed significantly to the worsening health of everyone who uses one.

And use one...we do. Research indicates that microwave ovens are fixtures in at least 90% of all homes and restaurants in America.

This is a particularly alarming statistic, but runs parallel to the understanding that everything reported to be good for you isn't.

WHAT'S SO PROBLEMATIC ABOUT MICROWAVING

If you can put aside the alleged convenience of a microwave oven, the science alone would make a clear thinking person refuse to use one.

The act of warming food or cooking is accomplished by introducing heat to the food being cooked. Fire does this just fine, but in the interest of technology, some genius (I'm being kind) decided that the use of a microwave tube to generate heat by disturbing the molecules of the item being cooked would be more efficient. Well, he was right about one thing. It was at least faster.

But, while the principles of this strategy actually work, it also works to destroy the molecules of your food. In other words, while it looks like you're eating broccoli, a steak, chicken, etc., the molecular composition is altered to a state that when you consume your food, that food interacts with the systems of your body in a manner that causes ill affects.

Let's look at what we actually know from the volumes of research done in this area.
- Placing plastic containers in the microwave or using plastic plates or covers made of plastic leach carcinogenic (cancer causing) toxics into your food when warmed or cooked in a microwave.
- Because of heat calibration problems, the food's temperature may elevate to levels that will cause explosions.

- It is recommended that you never warm a baby's milk in the microwave for two reasons;

  - The threat of exploding their glass bottles or leaching dangerous toxins into their milk from plastic bottles, and
  - The mircrowave destroys the disease fighting ability of breast milk

- The chemical structure of food warmed or cooked in a microwave oven changes (rendering the food void of its nutrients and even worse making the food poisonous to your system).
- Food prepared or cooked in a microwave oven changes the nutrients in the food in a way that changes your blood. The noted changes cause deterioration in human systems (as supported by research done in Switzerland by food scientist Hans Hertel).

In summary, what we don't know will hurt us. But a better approach is to honor accurate information (when it's presented and it has been) and make a better choice as a result.

RESOURCES/TOOLS THAT YOU CAN USE

I realized many years ago, that the old adage is true—you can't make someone do anything...even if it's right for them. However, it is my earnest wish that you throw your microwave away. This is one technological advance that did not do any of us well.

The reality though is that there is a product that can adequately replace your microwave and provide a way for you to prepare your food quickly. The difference is, there are no negative health impacts associated with the product.

It's called a convection oven. With this counter top appliance, you will be able to broil, bake, fry, roast, boil, and grill. It promotes low-fat cooking, and uses 80% less energy than standard ovens. Use this link http://sn.im/nu70g now. It will take you my A-Store—a site where I've partnered with Amazon to provide you with the options you need.

On the first page of that site, you will see three convection oven choices that will enable you to "feel no pain" when you throw your microwave away.

Tip No. 18

Oh Oh...Bottled Water...No No

In choosing the topics that are presented in this book, the central theme for each is its relevancy to your health; however, some (like this one) also affect world wellness.

What I mean in saying that is simple. Bottled water represents yet another technological advance given to us as a convenience yet there are problems that threaten personal health and the world's ecological systems.

Bottled Water: An Ecological Nightmare

Huge consumption = huge problems. Bottled water is a huge industry. According to statistics, worldwide consumption of bottled water doubled between 1997 and 2005. In America alone, the numbers indicate that 8.6 billion gallons of bottled water were consumed with sales increasing by 83% during this decade alone.

When you think about it and look backwards (for those of you over 30), could you have ever imagined during the 1970's that anyone would actually buy water in a plastic bottle?

Research indicates that it was a French company named Perrier that convinced people that it was cool to drink water out of bottle. And as they say, the rest is history. As the industry developed, the most cost effective container proved to be plastic. Once again, the rest is history.

Yes, it is an amazing thing to consider, but the statistics speak volumes.
- Plastic bottles in the United States require some 1.5 million barrels of oil to manufacture each year--enough to power 100,000 cars.
- Some 86% of plastic bottles in the United States never get recycled.
- Bottled water requires 2,000 times more energy to produce than it does to deliver tap water.
- Regarding impacts on landfill capacity, the Government's Accounting Office (GAO) found that about three-quarters of the water bottles produced in the United States in 2006 were discarded and not recycled.
- It takes a plastic water bottle 1,000 years before it starts to decompose.
- When burned, plastic water bottles release toxic smoke into the air and destroys the ozone layer that protects us from UV rays.
- When you throw your one or two plastic bottles in the garbage each day and think that it's no big deal consider this, your trashed bottles contribute to an estimated 37.5 billion plastic bottles that are not recycled in the US each year or 150 billion globally. If all of these bottles were lined up together they could stretch to the Moon and back 39 times. How's that for a super highway?

- Independent tests of bottled water indicate that chemical contamination has been found. While the source of the contamination (in many cases) could not be determined, it was not ruled out that the possible source of the contamination was the plastic containers in which the water was stored.

RESOURCES/TOOLS THAT YOU CAN USE

As noted in my report, "Change Your Water, Change Your Life", your best source of water is closer than you think.

Make your own utilizing a great filtration unit and alkalinize it as shown in the report alluded to above. Many of us enjoy having water available to us throughout the day. Store your water (preferably in glass containters). Pick up a copy of the report above and enjoy instantly improved health.

SOUL

TIP No. 19

Be Grateful or Show Gratitude

Webster's unabridged dictionary defines gratitude as the quality or feeling of being grateful or thankful.

As a result of the many recent published works on the natural laws of the universe ("The Secret" being the most popular among those works), more attention is now being given to qualities that had previously been discounted or judged as antiquated.

The qualities of humility, thankfulness and gratitude have a way of balancing you in a world that too easily will disparage those who demonstrate them by attaching such labels as weak, fragile or lacking toughness.

Truth is, the universe is a place that functions by rules that most of us would rather usurp. Since we are not by any standard equal to the universe, it is a better bet to exist in its harmony rather than oppose it.

So, count your blessings and acknowledge your very existence with gratitude. Take time (sometime during the day or evening) to do some deep breathing and reflect on those things that are good in your life (even those things that you take for granted like your health...that you can see...that you're able to smell...that you are able to walk, etc.). Express being grateful for all of the wonderful things in your life—especially the people who bring you joy and inspiration.

Think about this for a minute. Those of you who are parents know the sense of well being felt when your children show gratitude for those things that you've done for them. Your natural reaction is to do more for your children and provide that feeling for them more frequently. Now, while your expressions of gratitude should not be done with self-centered expectation, the universe has a way of granting gifts to those who are grateful for what it has already given them.

Living with gratitude opens your heart and makes life much more enjoyable. When you're ungrateful and resentful, you will be more stressed and pump out cortisol more often than normal.

Cortisol makes you fat, age prematurely and is associated with practically every disease known to man.

On the other hand, gratitude opens your heart and frees your mind.

TIP No. 20

Take Responsibility

I am famously known by my closet friends as someone who absolutely abhors people who shirk responsibility. In fact, I'm convinced that we've become a culture of people who would rather point a finger and look for a reason to blame someone else for everything than to accept ownership for our own indiscretions, frailties, inabilities, lack of judgment, etc.

We've become value-less.

It is easier to make it someone else's concern and then lie to yourself about how great you are than to take responsibility.

We need to stop this madness. We need to stop lying to ourselves. Most of us are unhealthy and miserable. We have become greedy in more ways than one. But as it relates to our physicality, the overweight reality that we accept as normal has most of us treading dangerously on the precipice of disease and even death.

The indicators are many. Here is a list of just a few...acid reflux, routine stomach aches, bloated stomachs, low back pains, poor self image, low self esteem, anxiety, headaches, depression, etc.

The reality is that we must only do one thing to break the cycle and begin a trip toward true health and wellness.

The one thing that must be done is simple; however, the step just might be too difficult for some to take. One must **take responsibility** for their current lot. The next step is to arm oneself with knowledge of how to right the wrong.

Your life becomes much more fulfilled when you take responsibility.

Being healthy and achieving wellness requires that you take responsibility and follow the knowledge that you discover even if it doesn't agree with the conventional path.

There are NO secrets or shortcuts, no diets or pills that will do anything for you except drain your pocketbooks and bank accounts.

Getting healthy, losing fat and living an awesome life boils down to taking complete responsibility for your life.

Take Responsibility

The alternative is an unhappy, unfulfilled life where an unfocused and irresponsible person meanders from one magic notion to yet another magic potion only to find oneself disappointed and never experiencing true "quality of life".

RESOURCES/TOOLS FOR YOU TO USE

This chapter presented the one-two punch. It is critical to be honest about what you see and who you see looking back at you in your mirror. More than anything else, this chapter was written to make you look at yourself and honestly take into account those things about yourself that you might not readily admit. Maybe it might be useful to make a list to identify those less than flattering qualities. After listing everything, write a plan of action to become better in that area. How about a plan to eradicate a shortcoming all together? If you can't empower yourself, find a professional in those areas and get the help you need. Re-read this chapter as many times as you need to. Honesty with self is pivotal if you seek to be better and become the authentic best that you can become. The next chapter will provide further insight.

TIP No. 21

Live "On Purpose"

Living on purpose is closely related to focus. It could actually be seen as focus but I felt that it should be included as its own section/chapter because of the exercises required to highlight how this is accomplished.

As it relates to my health and wellness, I evaluate how I'm doing on a daily basis. I find this to be a revealing and valuable exercise.

So, here are my early questions for you.

Is this necessary?

In your opinion, is there any value to doing this?

Truth is, if you are living your life on purpose then the answer to both questions is a resounding YES!

By living on purpose, I mean that you have established a plan and purpose for what you do, how you live and for how you go about doing what you do to be what and who you intend to be.

If you don't live with this level of focus, think about it.

Maybe that's the reason that you feel out of control at times.

For those of you who've said that you need to bring some order to your life, honest self-evaluation, self-accountability and the ability to devise a plan will bring about the order that you seek. You will even become inspired by noting your own progress. Reaching the small goals along the way usually is all the motivation necessary to throttle your continuance to your primary goals.

If you're challenged in the area of goal setting or if you're still fuzzy about a step by step process that will aide you in implementing goals the resource/tools section should give you the direction that you need.

RESOURCES/TOOLS FOR YOU TO USE
I was able to find a program that you can access online to supercharge your path toward making and achieving goals. Over the years, I've found that there's truth in what researchers have noted as the difference between those who succeed and those who don't. Simply put, those who succeed make a plan and carry it out. Maybe you feel that you need help in this area. If so, you can relax.

Live "On Purpose"

The program that I've found features breakthrough technology. It's accessible online and allows you to download the entire program onto your computer. This dynamic tool **will** help you to set and achieve your goals. To access the program for more information and/or to order it simply click or copy and paste the url into your browser: http://sn.im/jqv1y .

TIP No. 22

Make Your Loves and Friendships Vital, Vibrant and Meaningful

Not that I'm suggesting that you take an aloof pill or assume the personality of the most obnoxious person that you probably despise, but when was the last time that you gave any time to evaluating your friendships and love interests.

Oh...oh...yes, I did suggest that you evaluate your friendships and love interests.

I am not ashamed to confess that I know lots of people who are involved in toxic relationships. For those of you who aren't familiar with what I'm talking about or living in denial about this, those are the relationships that usually leave you drained when those people finally leave your presence. While in your presence though, they literally wreak havoc on your entire psyche. They seem to have the ability to effect you in the worst physical and emotional ways.

These people are usually self-centered, pushy, manipulative, inconsiderate, mean spirited or just plain mean. Okay, that represents the extreme. Maybe they are a little of all of the aforementioned. Regardless, their disposition, demeanor and behavior, the bottom line is that they grate you in all of the wrong ways.

My question is simple. Why is it that you tolerate them?

It might be a little difficult to pull away from some of these relationships because some of them are defined by obligation. But if your involvement is defined by obligation, you may consider that this obligatory affiliation has exhausted its usefulness.

That being said, in many instances though, there are a host of decisions that you can make to alter your tolerances and involvements with those people who personally drain you of your energy.

Accomplishing this is usually not as difficult as we make it. Your decision to develop new relationships with people who seek to live vibrantly seems to run the energy sappers away. Once again, your job (if you choose to accept it) is not to have a guilty conscious about the upgrade.

Understand me clearly. There are some people who need what you bring to them—even though they seem destined to the same rut that they seem to enjoy. It's a fine line. You will need to decide how much is enough.

Remember...it's difficult to avoid having your clothes soiled if you play by the ditch.

Tip No. 23

Valuing What's Important

Writing this chapter was actually more difficult than I first imagined because I am aware that there are varying perspectives of relevance as we consider valuing what's important.

Not that I am inclined to prove a point regarding perspectives, I'll offer a personal perspective in hopes that at least, you might find some direction.

For me, my journey back to health was extremely important. I am a former athlete. As such, I was proud, health conscious and always in the best of shape year round. I was rarely sick, hated taking medicine of any kind and consciously felt like a million dollars at all times.

But in those solitary moments, lying in the hospital as a 50-year old man wondering about what my life would become and how my health crisis would impact my future quality of life, I was scared and the prospects were daunting.

At this point, what could I do but plan to live to the best of my ability. The result of my face-to-face with self was my prioritizing the components of what I thought my future should look like and set about the task of pursuing that picture one step at a time.

Looking back at what I did, the steps were simple for me. Carrying them out; however, demanded that I remain focused on the desired results.

For many of you reading this, your story may not have life and death consequences; however, accomplishing your goal is equally relevant. This is personal. The importance is determined by you...not by someone else's scale of relevance. Be careful about guarding your important value.

I cannot emphasize enough that you understand completely that you and you only are the person who determines what's important and the relative value of that importance.

As examples...if it's important to you to have a higher paying job with commensurate responsibilities, you should not allow anyone or situations to destroy or prevent you from your mission. Remember, your accomplishment of this goal is important to you.

When you protect your mission and the steps taken along the way, you've given value to that goal. This mindset will sometimes mean that you have to become selfish with your time. It may mean being guarded about the conversations that you engage in or even the company that you keep.

Valuing What's Important

At this level of valuing what's important to you, those who are closest to you should understand your mission; however, in many cases they won't. Consequently, you need to understand, going in, that you will lose some along the way. If so, you also need to be alright with this. This will represent an opportunity for you to grow.

The hurt that you experience with those friends and family who would rather see you continue as you have in frustration are not worthy of hurt feelings if they can't accept your effort to do better for yourself. Keep it movin' and grow your life to its fullest potential.

Tip No. 24

Don't Become Obsessed with Possessions

You've heard the adage—The one who dies with the most toys wins.

Okay, let's examine and recognize this for the B.S. that it is.

No one cares about your toys. If you've elevated your collection of toys to god status, then those toys dominate your conversations and your life. Those possessions actually dehumanize you and have created an empty shell of shallowness.

That said, please understand that I am not saying that you should avoid the acquisition of toys or items that are nice, but do so in a balance that fosters your appreciation of the essence of your hard work and not as a symbol of "the trophy" that you display in a garish one-ups-man fashion.

I remember a discussion years ago with a group of aeronautic professionals that revolved around a rumored workforce reduction that all of us faced because the company that we worked for lost a significant contract.

I remember being amazed at how many of them were ruled by their possessions. Instead of the conversation revolving around life necessities, most were concerned about being able to make payments on possessions that they used to define the lifestyles that they acquired on the installment plan.

The other interesting note was that all of them lived way beyond their means. The example (for reference) is the guy making $75,000 a year but living the lifestyle of someone making at least $200,000 a year.

So, how does that happen? Better question is, why does that happen?

The why has to do with selling the perception to everyone he knows that "he's rolling", or he's made it to the big time. The how is done using credit cards and ill advised loans. In either case, it's bad news because now, your reason to go to work has everything to do with trying to pay for the debt created to support and maintain the illusion that you falsely created.

The better approach is to use your earned resources to create wealth through the increased value of your possessions--investments (not toys). You can then buy your toys using cash earned from your investments.

The bottom line is this: don't allow possessions to dominate any facet of your life. If you do, every day is a day of slavery to them.

Tip No. 25

Create a Vision Statement

This chapter was actually written months before I considered writing this book. It surfaced as the result of an assignment that I was doing in preparation for a sales meeting that I (as a team member of a very ineffective organization) had to attend.

Amid the backdrop of worldwide financial chaos, the management of the organization that I worked for at the time thought that leadership and self improvement exercises might magically create a better mindset among its workers and result in our abilities to overcome the obvious challenges of the economy and achieve despite everything that said it wouldn't happen.

To that, "we are going to transform ourselves and begin by developing personal vision statements," said our manager.

Well, at the outset, I, along with others in my office wanted no part of this. Everyone echoed thoughts that this would be another time consuming exercise that had nothing to do with producing sales.

What happened next; however, was pretty transformational.

The exercise didn't produce any sales. My sense though, was that my co-workers actually got a chance to evaluate who they were and what they wanted out of life while examining their personal motivations. Done correctly, this exercise forces you to pay attention to yourself in a way that may be a first for you.

So, for the record, the approach to their fashioning these esoteric statements was done in a rather irreverent way. I led the exercise. My co-workers had no idea what I was doing. They actually thought that I was about to do a stand up comedy routine.

I sat before them with a written report that I prepared the night before. I started into the report as if I were a news anchor. Adding further levity to the presentation, I started by stating my name and announcing that I approved this message (spoofing the political messages that were being aired in great volume at that time). It was at that point that I actually announced that my presentation was tied to a request by management for us to have our vision statements ready for presentation that day.

It was actually more than a bit funny at the time because I was the only one prepared. Once they realized what was going on, I could see that the group then split their focus between me and trying to write their own. Giving them some credit though, they did

Create A Vision Statement

listen well enough to write something that represented decent attempts to express respectable statements that were, at least, on point by definition.

So, what in the world is a vision statement and is there any value to completing this exercise? In truth, this is a useful tool if you're serious about self discovery and if you're committed to doing the work to propel yourself to the next level—whatever that may be.

So here it is. A vision statement is a vivid idealized description of a desired outcome that inspires, energizes and helps you create a mental picture of your target. It could be a vision of a part of your life, or the outcome of a project or goal.

Corporations routinely develop vision and mission statements. They're usually seen on wall plaques positioned prominently in their corporate offices.

For you though, this is about self discovery or owning up to who you are and what you're about.

In developing my statement, I read about an exercise where an instructor asked a group of professionals to create written vision statements that enabled them individually to finish the day having earned $10 dollars. After a few minutes, the group began to share their statements. Upon review, some seemed pretty good. In fact, some were very good. At the end of the exercise, the question was then asked, "Could any of those generate one million dollars?" The answer, per group consensus, was a resounding no.

So what's the point? You can't make a million dollars with a $10 dollar vision.

So how big is your vision?

It doesn't necessarily have to be big, but it should certainly be important to you.

Try these on for a look see.

Take the guy that we all know as Playa-Playa. You know him. He's cool, self absorbed, and actually reminds you of a pimp. He's a lady's man.

His vision statement might read something like this.

"I am the man...no ifs, ands, or buts," said while bouncing around like he's reacting to sharp pains in his legs.

At least it's short...albeit, very limited.

I find the next example to be more in line of what the exercise is all about.

Create A Vision Statement

"I have a dream that one day this nation will rise up and live out the true meaning of its creed: We hold these truths to be self-evident, that all men are created equal."
—Dr. Martin Luther King, Jr.

That vision statement was of particular interest at the time in that so much attention was being directed at the presidential election, where for the first time in the history of the United States, a black man ran for and won the highest elected position in the land-- President of these United States.

But as for me, I present my vision statement as one that crosses every fabric of my life. I work. I'm a father...a son...a brother...and a friend. Over the years of my life, I've done much and have seen plenty. I learned a lot and have endeavored to give more than I took.

In consideration of it all, the following words rolled off my tongue and through my lips with relative ease. I somehow had in mind the very thing that I'm doing today. I write about health and wellness in hopes of providing a base of information that will serve those in becoming better by the words and insight that I offer.

"My intention is to express the best of who I am (to those who might receive me) by providing a piece of what I've learned over the years and offering that as encouragement, inspiration, knowledge, motivation and solutions while sharing a few laughs along the way toward our next destination." —Gary Simms

Stay inspired and keep reaching.

BONUS

Who Else Wants to Grow Old Gracefully

GSimms, December 19, 2008
Modified Reprint: http://fyi-healthandwellness.blogspot.com
     www.Gsimms-HealthandWellness.com
     www.Article-Hangout.com

I can remember 'back in the day' (when I was a 20-something young stud) over hearing the conversations of the so-called 'ol folks' talking about growing old gracefully.

Well now I'm one of those 'ol folks' that I once looked at and said with a sense of youthful arrogance (actually foolishness) that their problems of aging would never be mine. As a 53-year old man, I'll share a secret with you—life happens. You busy yourself dealing with life's chores, challenges, and obstacles. You work, you raise a family, you create a home and along the way, you don't always make the best decisions regarding the maintenance of self. As a consequence, our bodies break down and more often than before suffer the ravages of illness and diminished function.

So, you do want to grow old gracefully don't you?   Well, how do you do that?

The secret is three-fold.

First, you should make sure that you're receiving optimum medical care. I recommend having a primary care medical team that includes a good general practice or family physician and an alternative medicine professional that is board certified in your state.

Oh…oh!!!!   What is this guy talking about.

Here's a dose of reality. Most physicians are trained to react to what you tell them about what hurts. Their role primarily is to prescribe medications to address the symptoms of your condition. Most alternative medicine physicians (Naturopathic Doctors—ND) are trained to identify those same conditions and prescribe protocols that might include herbs or other procedures to cure you of the problem that causes the symptom. Every situation is different so let me say that yours might be a curable condition but if it isn't and using the two medical professionals could make managing your situation more tolerable, then it's actually worth it to have this team in place.

By the way, it is absolutely imperative that these two professionals know of each other and support the work of each other as it relates to you.

Tip: Having one of the two refer you to the other would facilitate you receiving the best care from this scenario.

Who Else Wants to Grow Old Gracefully

Second, it is vital for your health that you follow a nutritional system that includes lots of fruit, vegetables, water, and healthy meat choices that don't include fried this and fried that.

Tip: Okay guys, this is for you as well. One of the programs that I like is the Weight Watchers program. Listen, when it comes to eating, you really think you know and don't need help, but this program is simple and gives you a road map that helps you eat in a healthy fashion. Their program is not about deprivation. Their program is all about assisting you in a lifestyle change related to how you deal with your nutritional intake. Trust me on this one. It works.

Last but not least…you've got to incorporate exercise in your lifestyle. It's not enough that you walk constantly at work. It's not enough that you periodically lift a few pounds of whatever during the day at work. You need a focused exercise program that includes both cardio (aerobic activity) and resistance training (anaerobic activity). This regimen will work best for you if you're doing it at least three times a week. For optimum results though, build your activity to five times a week.

Tip: There are so many devices and schemes being advertised to help you get in the 'shape of your life'. Don't fall for all the hype. You can become the best that you can be by following a simple plan that includes bodyweight exercises (only two movements to exercise the whole body—giving you both aerobic and anaerobic benefit) and 30-45 minutes of walking—aerobic benefit).

If you start slowly and build to the performance of this simple program for up to five days a week, you'll look in the mirror and want you kiss yourself in a few short weeks. Be patient though, nothing happens over night. I'm not going to have you believe that you will become Mr. or Ms. Olympia in six weeks; however in six weeks, you might pay a visit to someone that you haven't seen in a while only to have them not recognize you. Before starting your exercise program, you should pay a visit to your doctor and have him/her give you the stamp of approval to begin an exercise program.

To give you a little help on those two bodyweight exercises, check out this link: http://sn.im/jqz7j

There you will find an excellent program along with the details to help you get started and thrive along the way to great fitness at any age and from any starting point.

Good Luck!!!!!

Index/References

Focus: Pages 3-4
http://lifelearningtoday.com/2007/08/23/25-tips-to-become-more-productive-and-happy-at-work/;
http://liferemix.net/100-great-tips-improve-your-life;
www.Simpleology.com and Forum of the Healthy Urban Kitchen.

If What You Do For Work Is Not Your Passion, Find Your Passion & Do That: Pages 5-6
http://astore.amazon.com/gsimmshealth-20

Learn How to Manage or Eliminate Stress From Your Life: Pages 7-8
www.Self.com; The Complete Guide to Natural Healing; Journal of Health Psychology;
http://en.wikipedia.org/wiki/Music_Therapy;
http://stress.about.com/od/stresshealth/a/laughter. htm;

Learn The Skills Of Relaxation: Pages 9-12
http://www.councilforrelationships.org/articles/ stress-reduction-relaxation-meditation_6-28-04.htm;
http://www.mindtools.com/pages/article/ newTCS_05.htm

Develop A Thirst For Information and Knowledge: Pages 13-14
http://scienceblogs.com/notrocketscience/2009/07/why_information_is_its_own_reward__same_neurons_signal_thir.php;
http://www.knowledgehound.com/
http://en.wikipedia.org/wiki/Knowledge

If You're Motivated To Do Something, DO IT NOW: Pages 15-16
Psychology Today, August 2003;
http://en.wikipedia.org/wiki/Procrastination

Stop Accepting Advice From Everyone Wanting To Give It : Pages 17-18
http://dictionary.reference.com/

Make Fitness A Part Of Your Lifestyle : Pages 20-21

Become An Advocate Of Proper Nutrition : Pages 22-24
"Healthy Urban Kitchen Cookbook"

Eat Wholesome, Organic Plant Foods : Pages 25
JonTillman.com

Take A Metabolic Profile Test : Pages 26
http://www.naturalhealthyellowpages.com/metabolic/self_test.html

Change Your Drinking Water, Change Your Life : Pages 27-32
Water Institute of Japan, "Lessons from the Miracle Doctors", Alternative Health Information

Caution: Do Not Put That Toothpaste In Your Mouth : Pages 33-41
www.sci-toys.com, www.wikipedia.com, www.cosmeticdatabase.com

Eat 4-5 Meals A Day: Pages 42-44
http://www.fastweightlossidea.com, www.wtsp.com/pub/getfit/**meals**.doc, http://www.hss.gov.yk.ca/downloads/nutritiontips.pdf,http://www.snopes.com/medical/ myths/8glasses.asp, http://www.diagnose-me.com/ cond/C5223.html

Eat Grass Fed Beef, Free Range Chickens and Wild Caught Fish: Pages 45-48
http://www.americangrassfedbeef.com/grass-fed-natural-beef.asp, http://en.wikipedia.org/wiki/Fish_farming , http://www.time.com/time/health/article/0,8599,1663604,00.html, http://articles.mercola.com/sites/articles/archive/ 2003/05/10/farmed-salmon-part-one.aspx

No Ice Please: Pages 49-50
http://www.thatsfit.com/2007/12/06/restaurant-ice-cubes-dirtier-than-toilet-water/
http://www.msnbc.msn.com/id/13775964/

Throw Your Microwave Away: Pages 51-52
http://articles.mercola.com/sites/articles/archive/2003/11/05/microwave-food.aspx, NEXUS Magazine, Volume 2, #25 (April-May '95). The Hazards of Microwave Cooking--
http://www.mercola.com/article/microwave/hazards.htm

Oh Oh...Bottled Water...No No: Pages 53-55
http://abcnews.go.com/2020/Health/Story?id=728070&page=1, http://enewsusa.blogspot.com/2009/07/house-hearing-on-regulation-impacts-of.html, http://www.ehow. com/facts_4923034_facts-recycling-water-bottles.html

Be Grateful or Show Gratitude: Pages 56

Take Responsibility: Pages 57-58

Live "On Purpose": Pages 59-60
http://www.lifeonpurposeblog.com/

Make Your Loves & Friendships Vital, Vibrant and Meaningful : Pages 61

Valuing What's Important : Pages 62-63

Don't Become Obsessed With Possessions : Pages 64

Create a Vision Statement : Pages 65-67

Who Else Wants To Grow Old Gracefully : Pages 69-70